F. Paulsen and J. Waschke (eds.)

T0195467

Sobotta

Atlas of Anatomy

Learning Tables for Muscles, Joints and Nerves

Origin – Insertion – Innervation – Function

3rd Edition

English version with Latin nomenclature

Translated by
T. Klonisch and S. Hombach-Klonisch,
Winnipeg, Canada

ELSEVIER

Original Publication
Sobotta Lerntabellen Anatomie, 4. Auflage
© Elsevier GmbH, 2022.
All rights reserved.
ISBN 978-3-437-44160-8

This translation of Sobotta Lerntabellen Anatomie, 4th edition by Friedrich Paulsen and Jens Waschke was undertaken by Elsevier GmbH.

Elsevier GmbH, Bernhard-Wicki-Str. 5, 80636 Munich, Germany
We are grateful for any feedback and suggestions sent to: kundendienst@elsevier.com

The tables are also useful for an independent systematic learning and revision of subject matter.
Abbreviations: O = origin; I = insertion; F = function

ISBN 978-0-7020-6768-6

Adresses of the editors in chief
Prof. Dr. Friedrich Paulsen
Institute of Anatomy, Department of Functional and Clinical Anatomy
Friedrich Alexander University Erlangen-Nuremberg
Universitätsstraße 19
91054 Erlangen
Germany

Prof. Dr. Jens Waschke
Institute of Anatomy and Cell Biology, Department I
Ludwig-Maximilians-University (LMU) Munich
Pettenkoferstraße 11
80336 Munich
Germany

Bibliographical information of the Deutsche Nationalbibliothek
The Deutsche Nationalbibliothek has recorded this publication in the German National Bibliography; detailed bibliographic data are available on the internet at https://www.dnb.de

23   24   25   26   27   5   4   3   2   1

For copyright details for illustrations, see the credits for respective images.

Content strategist: Sonja Frankl
Project management: Dr. Andrea Beilmann, Sibylle Hartl
Editing and translating: Marieke O'Connor, Oxford, U.K.
Media rights management: Sophia Höver, Munich, Germany
Production management: Dr. Andrea Beilmann, Sibylle Hartl
Design: Nicola Kerber, Olching, Germany
Typesetting: abavo GmbH, Buchloe, Germany
Printing and binding: Drukarnia Dimograf Sp. z o. o., Bielsko-Biała, Poland
Cover design: Stefan Hilden, hilden_design, Munich; SpieszDesign, Neu-Ulm, Germany

Updated information is available on the internet at **www.elsevier.de**

Any errors?

 https://else4.de/978-0-7020-6768-6

We demand a lot from our contents. Despite every precaution it is still possible that an error can slip through or that the factual contents needs updating. For all relevant errors, a correction will be provided. With this QR code, quick access is possible.

We are grateful for each and every suggestion which could help us to improve this publication. Please send your proposals, praise and criticism to the following email address: kundendienst@elsevier.com

Table of content

Upper limb

Lower limb

Cranial nerves

Picture credits

The reference for all image sources in this work appears at the end of each figure legend in square brackets.
Explanation of the special characters:
[...-...] = work combined with illustrator

All unlabelled graphics and illustrations © Elsevier GmbH, Munich, Germany.
L126   Dr. med. Katja Dalkowski, Buckenhof, Germany
S700   Sobotta archive: Sobotta. Atlas der Anatomie des Menschen, various editions, Elsevier/Urban & Fischer

Head

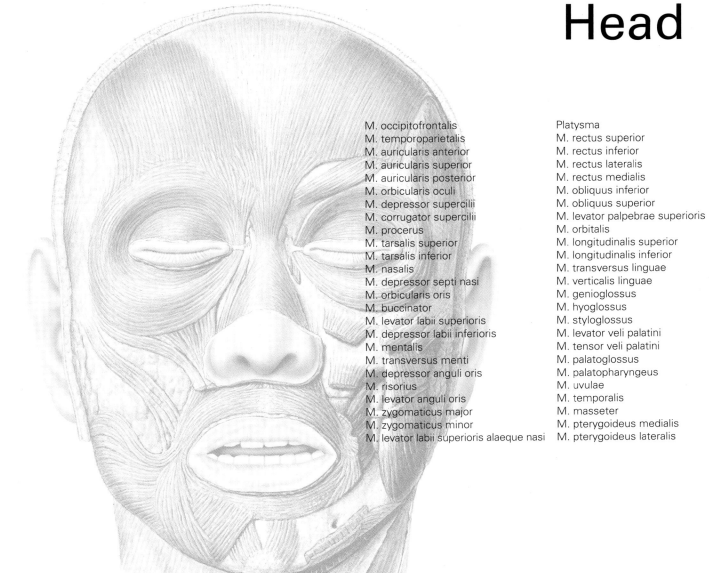

M. occipitofrontalis
M. temporoparietalis
M. auricularis anterior
M. auricularis superior
M. auricularis posterior
M. orbicularis oculi
M. depressor supercilii
M. corrugator supercilii
M. procerus
M. tarsalis superior
M. tarsalis inferior
M. nasalis
M. depressor septi nasi
M. orbicularis oris
M. buccinator
M. levator labii superioris
M. depressor labii inferioris
M. mentalis
M. transversus menti
M. depressor anguli oris
M. risorius
M. levator anguli oris
M. zygomaticus major
M. zygomaticus minor
M. levator labii superioris alaeque nasi

Platysma
M. rectus superior
M. rectus inferior
M. rectus lateralis
M. rectus medialis
M. obliquus inferior
M. obliquus superior
M. levator palpebrae superioris
M. orbitalis
M. longitudinalis superior
M. longitudinalis inferior
M. transversus linguae
M. verticalis linguae
M. genioglossus
M. hyoglossus
M. styloglossus
M. levator veli palatini
M. tensor veli palatini
M. palatoglossus
M. palatopharyngeus
M. uvulae
M. temporalis
M. masseter
M. pterygoideus medialis
M. pterygoideus lateralis

→ Table 1 Facial muscles

1 Facial muscles

The facial (mimic) muscles only partially originate from defined bony structures, but all insert into the skin.

1.1 Forehead, vertex, temple

M. occipitofrontalis and M. temporoparietalis are collectively named the M. epicranius.

M. occipitofrontalis
N. facialis [VII]

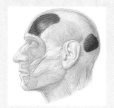

O: Venter frontalis: skin of the forehead
Venter occipitalis: Linea nuchalis suprema

I: Galea aponeurotica

F: forehead
Venter frontalis: wrinkling of the forehead (expression of surprise)
Venter occipitalis: smoothens wrinkles of the forehead

M. temporoparietalis
N. facialis [VII]

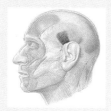

O: skin of the temple,
Fascia temporalis

I: Galea aponeurotica

F: moves the skin of the head downwards, tenses the Galea aponeurotica, although this is not a very distinct function

1.2 Auricle

M. auricularis anterior
N. facialis [VII]

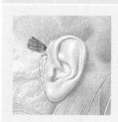

O: Fascia temporalis

I: at the front of the auricle

F: moves the auricle in a superior and anterior direction

M. auricularis superior
N. facialis [VII]

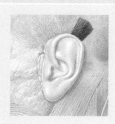

O: Galea aponeurotica

I: at the top of the auricle

F: moves the auricle in a superior and posterior direction

M. auricularis posterior
N. facialis [VII]

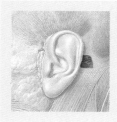

O: Proc. mastoideus

I: at the back of the auricle

F: moves the auricle in a posterior direction

1.3 Palpebral fissure

M. orbicularis oculi (surrounds the Aditus orbitae like a sphincter)
N. facialis [VII]

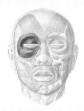

O: Pars orbitalis: Crista lacrimalis anterior, Proc. frontalis of the maxilla, Os lacrimale, Lig. palpebrale mediale
Pars palpebralis: Lig. palpebrale mediale
Pars lacrimalis (HORNER's muscle): Crista lacrimalis posterior of the Os lacrimale

I: Pars orbitalis: Lig. palpebrale laterale
Pars palpebralis: Lig. palpebrale laterale
Pars lacrimalis: lacrimal duct, palpebral fissures, posterior part of the Septum lacrimale

F: Pars orbitalis: powerful eyelid closure
Pars palpebralis: gentle eyelid closure, stabilises the lower eyelid; participates in blinking
Pars lacrimalis: induces a not yet fully understood pressure-suction mechanism, driving the lacrimal fluid via the Canaliculi lacrimales into the Saccus lacrimalis → stimulates the outflow of tears

M. depressor supercilii (separation of the Pars orbitalis of the M. orbicularis oculi)
N. facialis [VII]

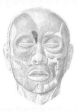

O: Pars nasalis of the Os frontale, dorsum of the nose

I: medial third of the skin of the eyebrow

F: lowers the skin of the eyebrow

M. corrugator supercilii
N. facialis [VII]

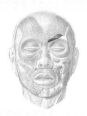

O: Pars nasalis of the Os frontale

I: middle third of the skin of the eyebrow

F: pulls the skin of the forehead and eyebrows towards the root of the nose, creates a vertical fold above the root of the nose (anger, thinking); supports the vigorous closure of the eyelid

M. procerus
N. facialis [VII]

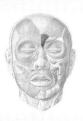

O: Os nasale

I: skin of the glabella

F: pulls the medial part of the eyebrow downwards, thereby inducing horizontal folds on the dorsum of the nose (wrinkling of the nose)

M. tarsalis superior (smooth muscles)
Sympathicus

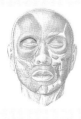

O: Tendon of the M. levator palpebrae superioris, structural support of the upper eyelid

I: Tarsus superior

F: widening of the palpebral fissure, vertical tightening of the upper eyelid

M. tarsalis inferior (smooth muscles)
Sympathicus

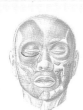

O: Structural support of the lower eyelid

I: Tarsus inferior

F: widening of the palpebral fissure, vertical tightening of the lower eyelid

1.4 Nose

M. nasalis
N. facialis [VII]

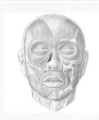

O: Pars alaris: maxilla at the level of the lateral incisor
Pars transversa: maxilla at the level of the canine

I: Pars alaris: nasal wing, rim of the nasal opening
Pars transversa: tendinous plate of the dorsum of the nose

F: moves the nasal wings and the nose
Pars alaris: dilates the nasal opening
Pars transversa: narrows the nasal opening (amazement, exhilaration)

M. depressor septi nasi
N. facialis [VII]

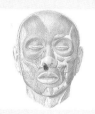

O: maxilla at the level of the medial incisor

I: Cartilago septi nasi

F: moves the nose downwards, dilates the nostrils

1.5 Mouth

M. orbicularis oris
N. facialis [VII]

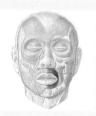

O: Pars marginalis and **Pars labialis:** lateral of the Angulus oris

I: skin of the lip

F: closes the lips, creates labial tension (of the lips)
Pars marginalis: pulls red part (vermilion) of the lips inwards
Pars labialis: pursing (pushing out) of the lips
→ Muscles of upper and lower lip can act independently
→ The muscle is used for food ingestion, articulation and facial expression

M. buccinator
N. facialis [VII]

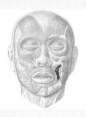

O: maxilla,
Raphe pterygomandibularis,
Mandibula

I: Angulus oris

F: tenses the lips, increases pressure within the oral cavity, e.g. during blowing and chewing, presses the cheeks against the teeth; prevents biting of the cheeks when chewing

M. levator labii superioris
N. facialis [VII]

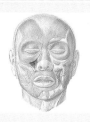

O: maxilla over the Foramen infraorbitale

I: upper lip

F: pulls the upper lip laterally upwards, dilates the nostrils (dissatisfaction, crying)

1.5 Mouth (continued)

M. depressor labii inferioris
N. facialis [VII]

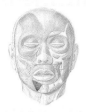

O: Mandibula below the Foramen mentale

I: lower lip

F: pulls the lower lip laterally downwards, purses the vermilion part of the lower lip (dislike)

M. mentalis
N. facialis [VII]

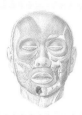

O: Mandibula, at the level of the lower lateral incisor

I: skin of the chin

F: creates chin dimple, everts and protrudes the lower lip (together with the M. orbicularis oris; 'a pout')

M. transversus menti
N. facialis [VII]

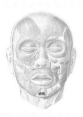

O: transverse separation from the M. mentalis

I: skin of the mental protuberance

F: moves the skin of the chin

M. depressor anguli oris
N. facialis [VII]

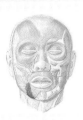

O: lower margin of the Mandibula

I: Angulus oris

F: moves the angle of the mouth downwards (discontent, grief)

M. risorius
N. facialis [VII]

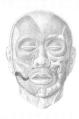

O: Fascia parotidea, Fascia masseterica

I: Angulus oris

F: broadens the mouth (grin), creates dimples

Head

1.5 Mouth (continued)

M. levator anguli oris
N. facialis [VII]

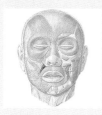

O: Fossa canina of the maxilla

I: Angulus oris

F: pulls the angle of the mouth medially upwards

M. zygomaticus major
N. facialis [VII]

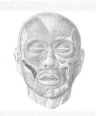

O: Os zygomaticum

I: Angulus oris

F: pulls the angle of the mouth laterally upwards (joy, muscle of laughter/smile)

M. zygomaticus minor
N. facialis [VII]

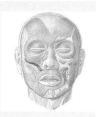

O: Os zygomaticum

I: Angulus oris

F: pulls the angle of the mouth laterally upwards

M. levator labii superioris alaeque nasi
N. facialis [VII]

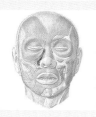

O: Proc. frontalis of the maxilla (medial orbital wall)

I: nasal wing, upper lip

F: lifts the lips and nasal wings (breathing through the nostrils; dissatisfaction, arrogance, disdain)

1.6 Neck

Platysma
N. facialis [VII]

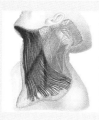

I: Basis mandibulae, Fascia parotidea

I: skin below the clavicle, Fascia pectoralis

F: tenses the skin of the neck, generates longitudinal folds, pulls the angle of the mouth laterally, promotes venous blood flow in the superficial cervical veins (fright, disgust)

Head

2 Extraocular muscles of the eyeball

M. rectus superior
N. oculomotorius [III], R. superior

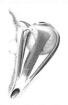

I: upper section of the Anulus tendineus communis

I: above, rostral to the equator on the eyeball

F: raises the visual axis, adducts and rotates the eyeball inward

M. rectus inferior
N. oculomotorius [III], R. inferior

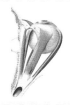

I: lower section of the Anulus tendineus communis

I: below, rostral to the equator on the eyeball

F: lowers the visual axis, adducts and rotates the eyeball outward

M. rectus lateralis
N. abducens [VI]

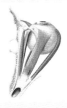

I: lateral section of the Anulus tendineus communis

I: lateral, rostral to the equator on the eyeball

F: abducts the eyeball

M. rectus medialis
N. oculomotorius [III], R. inferior

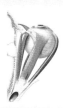

I: medial section of the Anulus tendineus communis

I: medial, rostral to the equator on the eyeball

F: adducts the eyeball

M. obliquus inferior
N. oculomotorius [III], R. inferior

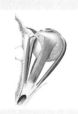

I: medial section of the orbital floor behind the orbital margin; on the maxilla lateral of the Sulcus lacrimalis

I: posterolateral quadrant of the eyeball

F: raises the visual axis, abducts and rotates the eyeball outward

M. obliquus superior
N. trochlearis [IV]

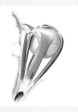

I: Corpus ossis sphenoidalis, above and medial to the Canalis opticus

I: posterolateral quadrant of the eyeball

F: lowers the visual field, abducts and rotates the eyeball inward

M. levator palpebrae superioris
N. oculomotorius [III], R. superior

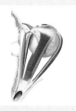

I: Ala minor ossis sphenoidalis, anterior to the Canalis opticus

I: front surface of the tarsus in the upper eyelid; fibres to the skin and to the Fornix conjunctivae

F: raises the upper eyelid

M. orbitalis (MÜLLER's muscle, smooth muscles)
Sympathicus

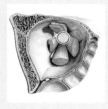

I: Periorbita below the Fissura infraorbitalis

I: Periorbita above the Fissura infraorbitalis

F: function not fully understood, springy abutmunt for the orbital content

3 Muscles of the tongue

3.1 Intrinsic muscles of the tongue (internal muscles)

M. longitudinalis superior
N. hypoglossus [XII]

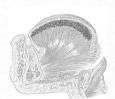

I: Radix linguae	**I:** Apex linguae	**F:** shortens and broadens the tongue, elevates the tip of the tongue

M. longitudinalis inferior
N. hypoglossus [XII]

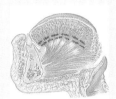

I: Radix linguae	**I:** Apex linguae	**F:** shortens and broadens the tongue, lowers the tip of the tongue

M. transversus linguae
N. hypoglossus [XII]

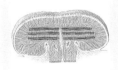

O: lateral margin of the tongue, Septum linguae	**I:** lateral margin of the tongue, Aponeurosis linguae	**F:** narrows the tongue and, in association with the M. verticalis linguae, extends the tongue

M. verticalis linguae
N. hypoglossus [XII]

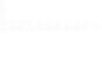

I: Radix linguae	**I:** Aponeurosis linguae	**F:** broadens the tongue

Head

3.2 Extrinsic muscles of the tongue (external muscles)

M. genioglossus
N. hypoglossus [XII]

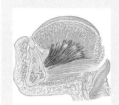

O: Spina mentalis of the Mandibula

I: Aponeurosis linguae

F: moves the tongue in an anterior and inferior direction, sticks the tongue out of the mouth

M. hyoglossus
N. hypoglossus [XII]

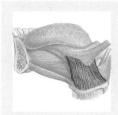

O: Cornu majus and Corpus ossis hyoidei

I: Aponeurosis linguae

F: moves the tongue in a posterior and inferior direction; its unilateral contraction lowers the tongue on the same side

M. styloglossus
N. hypoglossus [XII]

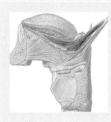

O: Proc. styloideus of the Os temporale

I: Aponeurosis linguae

F: moves the tongue in a posterior and superior direction; its unilateral contraction induces the tongue to move to the same side, with an inclination of the dorsum of the tongue to the opposite side

4 Muscles of the palate

M. levator veli palatini
Rr. pharyngeales of the N. glossopharyngeus [IX] and of the N. vagus [X] (= Plexus pharyngeus)

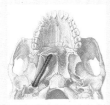

O: inferior surface of the petrous part of the Os temporale, Cartilago tubae auditivae

I: Aponeurosis palatina

F: elevates the soft palate, widens the lumen of the auditory tube

M. tensor veli palatini (is looped around the Hamulus ossis pterygoidei as a hypomochlion)
N. musculi tensoris veli palatini of the N. mandibularis [V/3]

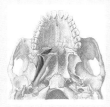

O: Fossa scaphoidea on the Proc. pterygoideus, membranous part and cartilage of the Tuba auditiva

I: Aponeurosis palatina

F: tenses the soft palate and widens the lumen of the auditory tube

M. palatoglossus
N. glossopharyngeus [IX]

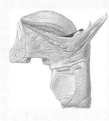

O: Aponeurosis palatina

I: radiates into the intrinsic muscles of the tongue, lateral margin of the Radix linguae

F: lowers the soft palate, simultaneously elevates the root of the tongue and thereby narrows the Isthmus faucium

M. palatopharyngeus
Plexus pharyngeus (N. glossopharyngeus [IX], N. vagus [X])

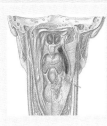

O: Aponeurosis palatina, Hamulus pterygoideus, Lamina medialis processus pterygoidei

I: lateral wall of the pharynx, upper margin of the thyroid cartilage

F: tenses the soft palate; pulls the pharyngeal wall in an anterior, superior and medial direction during swallowing; works together with the muscle on the opposite side

M. uvulae (unpaired muscle)
Rr. pharyngeales of the N. glossopharyngeus [IX] and of the N. vagus [X] (= Plexus pharyngeus)

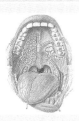

O: Aponeurosis palatina

I: stroma and tip of the Uvula palatina

F: shortens the Uvula palatina, thereby thickening it

5 Masticatory muscles

The M. masseter can be easily palpated through the skin along its course from the mandibular angle to the zygomatic arch. When clenching the teeth, the deep belly of the M. temporalis becomes noticeable in the temporal fossa. The M. pterygoideus medialis is located on the inner surface of the lower jaw (Ramus mandibulae). The M. pterygoideus lateralis projects anteriorly from the temporomandibular joint.

M. temporalis
Nn. temporales profundi (N. mandibularis [V/3])

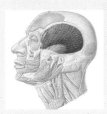

O: Os temporale inferior to the Linea temporalis inferior, deep lamina of the Fascia temporalis

I: Proc. coronoideus mandibulae

F: bilaterally:
- closes the jaws (strongest masticatory muscle) → adduction
- anterior part: pulls the mandible forward (= protrusion)
- posterior part: pulls the mandible backward (= retrusion)

unilaterally:
- on the working side: stabilisation of the Caput mandibulae (posterior part)
- balancing side: anterior shifting of the Caput mandibulae, rotation to the opposite (contralateral) side; the posterior part of the muscle keeps the Caput mandibulae in a resting position in the Fossa mandibulae

M. masseter
N. massetericus (N. mandibularis [V/3])

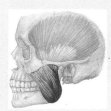

O: Pars superficialis: inferior margin of the Arcus zygomaticus
Pars profunda: inner surface of the Arcus zygomaticus

I: Pars superficialis: Angulus mandibulae (Tuberositas masseterica)
Pars profunda: inferior margin of the Mandibula

F: strong closure of the jaws (adduction)
Pars superficialis: pulls the mandible (Mandibula) forward (= protrusion)

M. pterygoideus medialis
N. pterygoideus medialis (N. mandibularis [V/3])

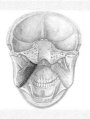

O: Fossa pterygoidea

I: inferior margin of the Mandibula (Tuberositas pterygoidea)

F: bilaterally:
- adduction of the mandible, protrusion of the mandible

unilaterally:
- grinding movement – on the balancing side: shifts the Caput mandibulae anteriorly and rotates to the opposite (contralateral) side

M. pterygoideus lateralis
N. pterygoideus lateralis (N. mandibularis [V/3])

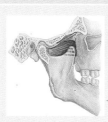

O: Caput superius: Crista infratemporalis of the Os sphenoidale
Caput inferius: Lamina lateralis of the Proc. pterygoideus

I: Caput superius: disc and capsule of the Articulatio temporomandibularis
Caput inferius: Proc. condylaris mandibulae (Fovea pterygoidea)

F: Caput superius:
- bilaterally: initiates the opening of the jaw by pulling the Discus articularis forward
- unilaterally: grinding movement – on the balancing side: shifts the Caput mandibulae forward

Caput inferius:
- bilaterally: fixes the Caput mandibulae to the tubercle slope during adduction
- unilaterally: grinding movement – on the working side: stabilises the resting condyle during the rotational movements

Neck

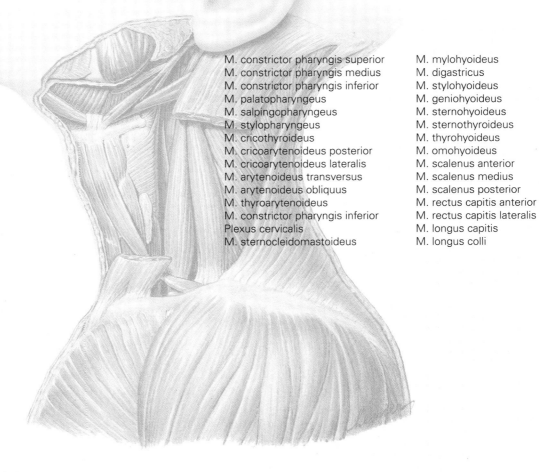

M. constrictor pharyngis superior
M. constrictor pharyngis medius
M. constrictor pharyngis inferior
M. palatopharyngeus
M. salpingopharyngeus
M. stylopharyngeus
M. cricothyroideus
M. cricoarytenoideus posterior
M. cricoarytenoideus lateralis
M. arytenoideus transversus
M. arytenoideus obliquus
M. thyroarytenoideus
M. constrictor pharyngis inferior
Plexus cervicalis
M. sternocleidomastoideus

M. mylohyoideus
M. digastricus
M. stylohyoideus
M. geniohyoideus
M. sternohyoideus
M. sternothyroideus
M. thyrohyoideus
M. omohyoideus
M. scalenus anterior
M. scalenus medius
M. scalenus posterior
M. rectus capitis anterior
M. rectus capitis lateralis
M. longus capitis
M. longus colli

Neck

6 Muscles of the pharynx

The pharyngeal muscles are divided into constrictor muscles (Mm. constrictores pharyngis superior, medius and inferior) and levator muscles (M. stylopharyngeus, M. salpingopharyngeus and M. palatopharyngeus).

6.1 Pharyngeal constrictor muscles

M. constrictor pharyngis superior
Rr. pharyngeales of the N. glossopharyngeus [IX] (= Plexus pharyngeus)

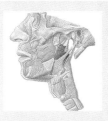

O: Pars pterygopharyngea: Lamina medialis of the Proc. pterygoideus, Hamulus ossis pterygoidei
Pars buccopharyngea: Raphe pterygomandibularis
Pars mylopharyngea: Linea mylohyoidea of the Mandibula
Pars glossopharyngea: M. transversus linguae

I: Membrana pharyngobasilaris, Raphe pharyngis

F: participation in swallowing, narrows the pharyngeal space (PASSAVANT's ridge), separates the epipharynx from the mesopharynx

M. constrictor pharyngis medius
Rr. pharyngeales of the N. glossopharyngeus [IX] and of the N. vagus [X] (= Plexus pharyngeus)

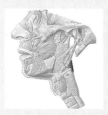

O: Pars chondropharyngea: Cornu minus ossis hyoidei
Pars ceratopharyngea: Cornu majus ossis hyoidei

I: Raphe pharyngis

F: participation in swallowing, narrows the pharyngeal space from behind, promotes wave-like contractions running downwards to support the transport of ingested food into the oesophagus (peristalsis)

M. constrictor pharyngis inferior
Rr. pharyngeales of the N. vagus [X] (= Plexus pharyngeus)

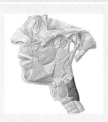

O: Pars thyropharyngea: Cartilago thyroidea
Pars cricopharyngea: lateral side of the Cartilago cricoidea

I: Raphe pharyngis

F: closes the Aditus laryngis by elevating the larynx, narrows the pharyngeal space from behind, promotes wave-like downward contractions to support the transport of ingested food into the oesophagus (peristalsis)

6.2 Pharyngeal levator muscles

M. palatopharyngeus (functionally also belonging to the palatine muscles)
Rr. pharyngeales of the N. glossopharyngeus [IX] (= Plexus pharyngeus)

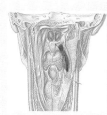

O: Aponeurosis palatina, Hamulus pterygoideus, Lamina medialis processus pterygoidei

I: lateral wall of the pharynx, upper margin of the thyroid cartilage

F: tenses the soft palate; pulls the pharyngeal wall in an anterior, superior and medial direction during swallowing; works together with the muscle on the opposite (contralateral) side

M. salpingopharyngeus
Rr. pharyngeales of the N. glossopharyngeus [IX] (= Plexus pharyngeus)

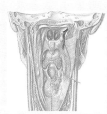

O: Cartilago tubae auditivae

I: projects into the lateral wall of the pharynx

F: elevates the pharynx, opens the Tuba auditiva; works together with the muscle on the opposite (contralateral) side

M. stylopharyngeus
R. musculi stylopharyngei of the N. glossopharyngeus [IX]

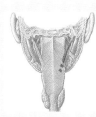

O: Proc. styloideus of the Os temporale

I: Cartilago thyroidea, projects into the lateral wall of the pharynx

F: elevates the pharynx, pulls the pharyngeal wall upwards above the bolus; its horizontally oriented fibre bundles dilate the Isthmus faucium; works together with the muscle on the opposite (contralateral) side

Neck

7 Muscles of the larynx

M. cricothyroideus (Anticus) (Pars recta: superficial, Pars obliqua: deep, Pars interna: deep)
R. externus of the N. laryngeus superior of the N. vagus [X]

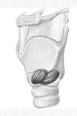

O: Pars interna: ventral surface of the lamina of Cartilago cricoidea
Pars recta and **Pars obliqua:** ventral surface of the lamina of the Cartilago cricoidea

I: inner surface of the lamina of the Cartilago thyroidea and Conus elasticus
Pars recta: inferior margin of the lamina of the Cartilago thyroidea
Pars obliqua: Cornu inferius of the Cartilago thyroidea

F: tenses (elongates) the vocal ligaments by tilting the cricoid cartilage (strongest tensor muscle of the vocal ligaments → gross tension)

M. cricoarytenoideus posterior (Posticus)
N. laryngeus recurrens of the N. vagus [X]

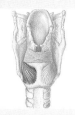

O: posterior surface of the lamina of Cartilago cricoidea

I: Proc. muscularis of the Cartilago arytenoidea

F: widens the glottis by lateral movement of the Proc. vocalis of the Cartilago arytenoidea and lateral tilt of the Cartilago arytenoidea

M. cricoarytenoideus lateralis (Lateralis)
N. laryngeus recurrens of the N. vagus [X]

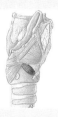

O: lateral upper margin of the Arcus of Cartilago cricoidea

I: Proc. muscularis of the Cartilago arytenoidea

F: closes the Pars intermembranacea of the glottis by medial (inward) rotation and slight elevation of the Cartilago arytenoidea, opens the Pars intercartilaginea for whispering ('whispering triangle')

M. arytenoideus transversus
N. laryngeus recurrens of the N. vagus [X]

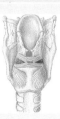

O: lateral rim and posterior surface of the Cartilago arytenoidea

I: lateral rim and posterior surface of the contralateral Cartilago arytenoidea

F: closes the Pars intercartilaginea of the glottis by inducing convergence of both of the Cartilago arytenoidea

M. arytenoideus obliquus
N. laryngeus recurrens of the N. vagus [X]

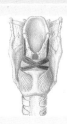

O: base of the posterior surface of the Cartilago arytenoidea
Pars aryepiglottica: tip of the Cartilago arytenoidea

I: tip of the contralateral Cartilago arytenoidea
Pars aryepiglottica: lateral margin of the Cartilago epiglottica

F: pulls the Cartilago arytenoidea medially, thereby narrowing the Pars intercartilaginea of the glottis and the entrance to the larynx, with subtle opening of the Pars intermembranacea

M. thyroarytenoideus
N. laryngeus recurrens of the N. vagus [X]

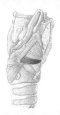

O: Pars externa: inner surface of the lamina of Cartilago thyroidea

I: Proc. muscularis and anterior surface of the Cartilago arytenoidea

F: closes the Pars intermembranacea of the glottis by moving next to and lowering the Proc. vocalis

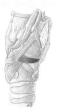

O: Pars thyroepiglottica: inner surface of the lamina of Cartilago thyroidea

I: lateral margin of the epiglottis and Plica vestibularis

F: narrows the entrance to the larynx

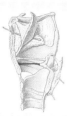

O: Pars interna (M. vocalis): the inside of the trigone of the Cartilago thyroidea, in the caudal third above the vocal ligament (tendon of BROYLES)

I: Portio thyrovocalis: Proc. vocalis, Portio thyromuscularis: Fovea oblonga

F: isotonic contraction:
- closes the Pars intermembranacea of the glottis by elongation or shortening of the vocal folds
isometric contraction:
- regulates tension of the vocal folds (fine-tuning) → regulates the oscillating part of the vocal folds

M. constrictor pharyngis inferior
Rr. pharyngeales of the N. vagus [X] (= Plexus pharyngeus)

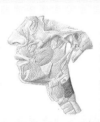

O: Pars thyropharyngea: lateral margin of the Cartilago thyroidea

I: Raphe pharyngis

F: elevates the larynx during swallowing, tenses the vocal folds, → Tab. 6 Muscles of the pharynx

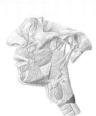

O: Pars cricopharyngea: posterior part of the outer surface of the Cartilago thyroidea

I: Raphe pharyngis

F: relaxes the vocal folds (debatable), → Tab. 6 Muscles of the pharynx

8 Branches and innervation areas of the Plexus cervicalis

	Motor	Sensory
Ansa cervicalis profunda Radix superior (= Radix anterior) Radix inferior (= Radix posterior)	Mm. infrahyoidei	
Rr. musculares	M. longus colli, M. longus capitis, Mm. recti capitis anterior and lateralis, Mm. intertransversarii anteriores cervicis, M. trapezius, M. levator scapulae, Mm. scaleni, M. geniohyoideus	
Branches of the Punctum nervosum (ERB's point) N. auricularis magnus		skin of the upper neck region, at the mandibular angle, anterior and posterior to the auricle, the major part of the auricle
N. transversus colli		skin in the upper anterior neck region
N. occipitalis minor		skin in the occipital region
Nn. supraclaviculares mediales, intermedii and laterales		skin in a line inferior to the clavicle
N. phrenicus	diaphragm	Pleura parietalis, pericardium, peritoneum

9 Lateral muscle of the neck

The M. sternocleidomastoideus derives from the same primordium as the M. trapezius (identical innervation). From its origin at the Proc. mastoideus it runs obliquely in an anterior, inferior and medial direction, and is integrated in the Lamina superficialis of the Fascia cervicalis.

M. sternocleidomastoideus
N. accessorius [XI]; Plexus cervicalis

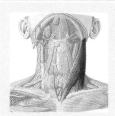

O: Caput sternale: ventral aspect of the sternum
Caput claviculare: sternal third of the clavicle

I: Proc. mastoideus, lateral Linea nuchalis superior

F: unilaterally active:
- turns the head to the contralateral side and inclines the head to the same side

bilaterally active:
- erects the head, bends the cervical spine
- auxiliary breathing muscle when the head is in a fixed position

10 Suprahyoid muscles

The suprahyoid muscles form the floor of the oral cavity and are antagonists of the infrahyoid muscles. The Venter anterior of the M. digastricus is located superficially. As a broad muscular plate, the M. mylohyoideus closes the oral cavity caudally. Inside, the rounded tract of the M. geniohyoideus lies against it. The Venter posterior of the M. digastricus and the M. stylohyoideus lie dorsally.

M. mylohyoideus (Both muscles on the right and left side together form a muscular plate that confines the oral cavity caudally.)
N. mylohyoideus (N. mandibularis [V/3])

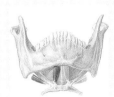

O: Linea mylohyoidea of the Mandibula

I: Raphe mylohyoidea, Corpus ossis hyoidei

F: bilaterally with fixed mandible:
- elevation of the hyoid bone during swallowing

bilaterally:
- depression of the mandible (opening the mouth) with a fixed hyoid bone
- elevation of the hyoid bone with fixed mandible during swallowing

unilaterally:
- grinding movement – ipsilateral rotation with fixed hyoid bone

M. digastricus (Venter posterior and Venter anterior are connected by an intermediate round tendon, which is fixed at the Cornu minus of the Os hyoideum.)
Venter anterior: N. mylohyoideus (N. mandibularis [V/3]);
Venter posterior: R. digastricus (N. facialis [VII])

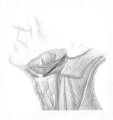

O: Incisura mastoidea of the Os temporale

I: Fossa digastrica of the Mandibula

F: bilaterally with fixed mandible:
- elevation of the hyoid bone during swallowing

Venter anterior:
- bilaterally: abduction of the mandible (opening the mouth) with fixed hyoid bone
- unilaterally: grinding movement – on the balancing side: shifts the Caput mandibulae anteriorly, with ipsilateral rotation

M. stylohyoideus
R. stylohyoideus (N. facialis [VII])

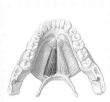

O: Proc. styloideus of the Os temporale

I: Corpus ossis hyoidei with two muscular bundles which encompass the intermediate tendon of the M. digastricus

F: bilaterally:
- elevation of the hyoid bone backwards during swallowing

M. geniohyoideus (right and left parts of the muscle lie close to each other – only separated by a thin septum of connective tissue)
Rr. ventrales aus C1–C2

O: Spina mentalis of the Mandibula

I: Corpus ossis hyoidei

F: bilaterally with a fixed hyoid bone:
- abduction of the mandible (opening the mouth)

unilaterally with fixed hyoid bone:
- grinding movement – ipsilateral rotation

bilaterally with fixed mandible:
- shifts the hyoid bone anteriorly and upwards

Neck

11 Infrahyoid muscles

The infrahyoid muscles are antagonists of the suprahyoid muscles. Located beneath the superficial M. sternohyoideus are the M. sternothyroideus and the M. thyrohyoideus. The course of the M. omohyoideus is the furthest to the lateral side.

M. sternohyoideus
Ansa cervicalis (Plexus cervicalis)

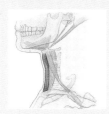

O: inner surface of the Manubrium sterni, joint capsule of the sternoclavicular articulation, Pars sternalis of the Clavicula

I: Corpus ossis hyoidei

F: pulls the hyoid bone caudally; in the case of isometric contraction fixes the hyoid bone for opening of the jaws and grinding movements

M. sternothyroideus
Ansa cervicalis (Plexus cervicalis)

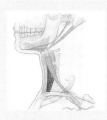

O: inner surface of the Manubrium sterni, costal cartilage of ribs 1 and 2

I: Linea obliqua of the lamina of the Cartilago thyroidea, Tuberculum superius and Tuberculum inferius of the Cartilago thyroidea

F: pulls the larynx caudally; in the case of isometric contraction fixes the larynx during phonation

M. thyrohyoideus
Ansa cervicalis (Plexus cervicalis)

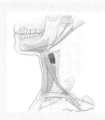

O: outer surface of the lamina of the Cartilago thyroidea, Tuberculum superius and Tuberculum inferius

I: Corpus ossis hyoidei and Cornu majus ossis hyoidei

F: pulls the hyoid bone and the larynx towards each other, raises the larynx (act of swallowing) with a fixed hyoid bone, lowers the hyoid bone with a fixed larynx and thereby affects phonation

M. omohyoideus (The Venter inferior and Venter superior are connected via an intermediate tendon which is attached to the Vagina carotica.)
Ansa cervicalis (Plexus cervicalis)

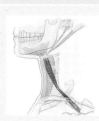

O: Venter inferior: Margo superior of the scapula, base of the Proc. coracoideus

I: Venter superior: Corpus ossis hyoidei

F: tenses the fascia of the neck, as the intermediate tendon is fused with the Vagina carotica, keeps the lumen of the V. jugularis interna open, pulls the hyoid bone caudally, and fixes the hyoid bone

12 Scalene muscles

The three scalene muscles, M. scalenus anterior, M. scalenus medius, and M. scalenus posterior, run to the upper ribs and form a triangular muscular plate at the lateral aspect of the cervical spine. The brachial plexus and the subclavian artery pass through the scalene triangle, delineated by the Mm. scaleni anterior and medius.

M. scalenus anterior
Direct branches of the Plexus cervicalis and Plexus brachialis

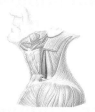

O: Tubercula anteriora of the Procc. transversi of the cervical vertebrae C3–C6

I: Tuberculum musculi scaleni anterioris of rib 1

F: the spinal column supports:
- bilaterally: elevates rib 1 and thereby the thorax (breathing muscle: inspiration)

the thorax supports:
- bilaterally: bending the spinal column
- unilaterally: lateral flexion of the spinal column to the same side, rotation to the other side

M. scalenus medius
Direct branches of the Plexus cervicalis and Plexus brachialis

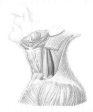

O: Tubercula of the Procc. transversi of the cervical vertebrae C3–C7

I: rib 1 posterior to the Sulcus arteriae subclaviae

F: the spinal column supports:
- bilaterally: enables ventral flexion of the neck, elevates rib 1 and thereby the thorax (breathing muscle: inspiration)

the thorax supports:
- unilaterally: lateral flexion of the spinal column to the same side

M. scalenus posterior
Direct branches of the Plexus cervicalis and Plexus brachialis

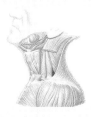

O: Tubercula posteriora of the Procc. transversi of the cervical vertebrae C5 and C6

I: rib 2

F: the spinal column supports:
- bilaterally: elevates ribs 2 and 3 and thereby the thorax (breathing muscle: inspiration)

the thorax supports:
- unilaterally: slight inclination of head

Neck

13 Prevertebral muscles

The prevertebral muscles are located to the right and left sides of the vertebral bodies of the cervical and upper thoracic vertebral column and are covered by the Lamina prevertebralis of the Fascia cervicalis. The M. rectus capitis anterior and M. rectus capitis lateralis connect the anterior and lateral parts of the atlas and axis.

M. rectus capitis anterior and M. rectus capitis lateralis
Direct branches of the Plexus cervicalis

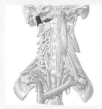

O: Proc. transversus and Massa lateralis of the atlas

I: Pars basilaris of the Os occipitale

F: bend the head ventrolaterally, turn the head to the ipsilateral side, inclination to the side (lateral flexion) of the head, fine-tuning in the head joints

M. longus capitis
Direct branches of the Plexus cervicalis

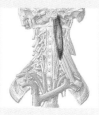

O: Tubercula anteriora of the Procc. transversi of the cervical vertebrae C3–C6

I: Pars basilaris of the Os occipitale

F: inclines the head ventrally, turns the head to the ipsilateral side, inclines the head to the side (lateral flexion)

M. longus colli
Direct branches of the Plexus cervicalis

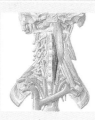

O: body of the fifth cervical to third thoracic vertebrae, Tubercula anteriora of the Procc. transversi of the cervical vertebrae C2–C5

I: Procc. transversi of the cervical vertebrae C5 and C6, body of the cervical vertebrae C2–C4, Tuberculum anterius of the atlas

F: inclines the head ventrally, turns the head to the ipsilateral side, inclines the head to the side (lateral flexion)

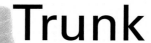

Trunk

Mm. intercostales externi
Mm. intercostales interni
Mm. intercostales intimi
Mm. subcostales
M. transversus thoracis
M. rectus abdominis
M. pyramidalis
M. obliquus externus abdominis
M. obliquus internus abdominis
M. transversus abdominis
M. cremaster
M. quadratus lumborum
M. serratus posterior superior
M. serratus posterior inferior
M. iliocostalis lumborum
M. iliocostalis thoracis
M. iliocostalis cervicis
M. longissimus thoracis
M. longissimus cervicis
M. longissimus capitis
Mm. intertransversarii laterales lumborum
Mm. intertransversarii mediales lumborum
Mm. intertransversarii thoracis
Mm. intertransversarii posteriores cervicis
Mm. intertransversarii anteriores cervicis

M. splenius cervicis
M. splenius capitis
Mm. levatores costarum
Mm. interspinales lumborum
Mm. interspinales thoracis
Mm. interspinales cervicis
M. spinalis thoracis
M. spinalis cervicis
M. spinalis capitis
Mm. rotatores
Mm. multifidi
M. semispinalis thoracis
M. semispinalis cervicis
M. semispinalis capitis
M. rectus capitis posterior major
M. rectus capitis posterior minor
M. obliquus capitis superior
M. obliquus capitis inferior
Diaphragma
M. levator ani
M. ischiococcygeus
M. transversus perinei profundus
M. sphincter urethrae externus
M. transversus perinei superficialis
M. ischiocavernosus
M. bulbospongiosus
M. sphincter ani externus

Trunk

14 Muscles of the thoracic wall

The M. pectoralis major shapes the surface of the anterior upper thoracic wall. Beneath this muscle lies the M. pectoralis minor. These two muscles, together with the M. subclavius, belong to the group of ventral muscles of the shoulder girdle (→ Tab. 26).

The Mm. intercostales externi and interni fill the intercostal spaces. The Mm. subcostales and the M. transversus thoracis lie next to them on the inner side of the thoracic wall.

Mm. intercostales externi
Nn. intercostales (Nn. thoracici)

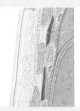

O: inferior costal margin from the Tuberculum costae to the bone-cartilage junction

I: superior costal margin of the next caudal rib

F: lift the ribs, inspiration

Mm. intercostales interni (The Mm. intercostales intimi are delineated on their inner side by the Vasa intercostalia posteriora and the N. intercostalis.)
Nn. intercostales (Nn. thoracici)

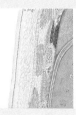

O: superior costal margin ventrally of the Angulus costae

I: inferior costal margin of the next cranial rib

F: depress the ribs, expiration

Mm. intercostales intimi (innermost part of the Mm. intercostales interni, frequently also called Mm. intercostales intimi)
Nn. intercostales (Nn. thoracici)

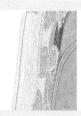

O: superior costal margin ventrally of the Angulus costae

I: inferior costal margin of the next cranial rib

F: depress the ribs, expiration

Mm. subcostales (inconstant muscles)
Nn. intercostales (Nn. thoracici)

O: superior margin of the lower ribs between the Tuberculum and Angulus costae

I: inferior margin of the lower ribs, skipping one rib

F: depress the ribs, expiration

M. transversus thoracis
Nn. intercostales (Nn. thoracici)

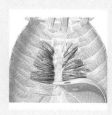

O: dorsally at the Corpus sterni and Proc. xiphoideus

I: Cartilago costalis of ribs 2–6

F: tenses the thoracic wall, expiration

15 Ventral muscles of the abdominal wall

The muscles of the anterior abdominal wall, the M. rectus abdominis and the M. pyramidalis, are located within the rectus sheath.

M. rectus abdominis
Nn. intercostales (Nn. thoracici)

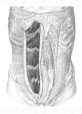

O: outer surface of the Cartilago costalis of ribs 5–7, Ligg. costoxiphoidea

I: Symphysis pubica

F: bends the torso, abdominal press, expiration (diaphragmatic or abdominal breathing type)

M. pyramidalis (inconstant muscle)
Caudal Nn. intercostales (Nn. thoracici)

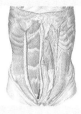

O: Symphysis pubica ventral to the M. rectus abdominis

I: Linea alba

F: 'tenses the Linea alba'

16 Lateral muscles of the abdominal wall

The M. obliquus externus abdominis, the M. obliquus internus abdominis and the M. transversus abdominis are collectively named the lateral muscles of the abdominal wall. Their tendinous plates form the rectus sheath. In both men and women, the M. cremaster separates from the M. obliquus abdominis internus and the M. transversus.

M. obliquus externus abdominis
Caudal Nn. intercostales (Nn. thoracici)

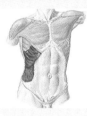

O: outer surface of ribs 5–12

I: Labium externum of the Crista iliaca, Lig. inguinale, participates in the formation of the anterior lamina of the rectus sheath

F: unilaterally active:
• rotates the thorax to the contralateral side
• bends the spinal column to the ipsilateral side
bilaterally active:
• bends the torso
• abdominal press
• expiration (diaphragmatic breathing type)

M. obliquus internus abdominis
Caudal Nn. intercostales (Nn. thoracici); N. iliohypogastricus; N. ilioinguinalis (Plexus lumbalis)

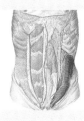

O: Fascia thoracolumbalis (deep layer), Linea intermedia of the Crista iliaca, Lig. inguinale

I: inferior margin of the Cartilago costalis of ribs 9–12, contributes to the anterior and posterior laminae of the rectus sheath above the Linea arcuata, below which all tendinous fibres project into the anterior lamina

F: unilaterally active:
• rotates the thorax to the ipsilateral side
• bends the spinal column to the ipsilateral side
bilaterally active:
• bends the torso
• abdominal press
• expiration (diaphragmatic breathing type)

M. transversus abdominis
Caudal Nn. intercostales (Nn. thoracici); N. iliohypogastricus; N. ilioinguinalis (Plexus lumbalis); N. genitofemoralis

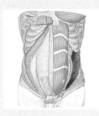

O: inner surface of the Cartilago costalis of ribs 7–12, Fascia thoracolumbalis (deep layer), Labium internum of the Crista iliaca, Lig. inguinale

I: contributes to the posterior lamina of the rectus sheath above the Linea arcuata, below which it contributes to the formation of the anterior lamina

F: abdominal press, expiration (diaphragmatic breathing type)

M. cremaster
N. genitofemoralis

O: separation of the M. obliquus internus and the M. transversus abdominis

I: surrounds the spermatic cord, in women the Lig. teres uteri

F: lifts the testis

17 Dorsal muscles of the abdominal wall

The M. quadratus lumborum forms the muscular basis of the posterior abdominal wall. The M. psoas major follows medially thereof.

M. quadratus lumborum
Caudal Nn. intercostales; Rr. musculares (Plexus lumbalis)

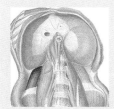

O: Labium internum of the Crista iliaca

I: rib 12, Proc. costalis of the lumbar vertebrae L4–L1

F: bends the spinal column to the ipsilateral side

18 Spinocostal muscles

The spinocostal muscles, M. serratus posterior superior and M. serratus posterior inferior, are thin muscles of minor functional relevance and are located deeply on the autochthonous muscles of the back.

M. serratus posterior superior
Cranial Nn. intercostales (Nn. thoracici)

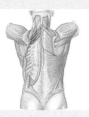

O: Proc. spinosus of the cervical vertebrae C6 and C7 and the thoracic vertebrae T1 and T2

I: ribs 2–5 lateral to the Angulus costae

F: elevates the ribs, inspiration

M. serratus posterior inferior
Caudal Nn. intercostales (Nn. thoracici)

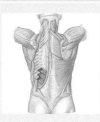

O: Proc. spinosus of the thoracic vertebrae T11 and T12 and the lumbar vertebrae L1 and L2

I: caudal margin of ribs 9–12

F: depresses ribs 9–12, also active during forced inspiration as an antagonist to the diaphragm

19 Autochthonous muscles of the back

19.1 Lateral tract

The lateral tract of the autochthonous muscles of the back covers the medial tract in the cervical and lumbar regions. Hence, it is also referred to as the superficial part of the autochthonous muscles of the back. The M. iliocostalis, the M. longissimus and the Mm. intertransversarii constitute the group of straight muscles. Diverging cranially in an oblique angle (spinotransversal) are the Mm. splenii.

The Mm. levatores costarum run in an oblique laterocaudal direction to the ribs.

a Sacrospinal system

M. iliocostalis lumborum
Rr. posteriores of the Nn. lumbales

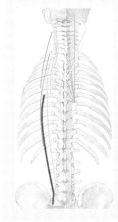

O: along with the M. longissimus thoracis from:
Labium externum of the Crista iliaca,
Facies dorsalis of the Os sacrum,
Fascia thoracolumbalis

I: Angulus costae of ribs 12–5

F: unilaterally active:
- lateroflexion
bilaterally active:
- extension
- braces the spinal column

M. iliocostalis thoracis
Rr. posteriores of the Nn. thoracici

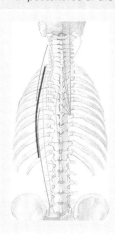

O: ribs 12–7 medial to the Angulus costae

I: Angulus costae of ribs (6) 7–1

F: unilaterally active:
- lateroflexion
bilaterally active:
- extension
- braces the spinal column

M. iliocostalis cervicis
Rr. posteriores of the Nn. cervicales

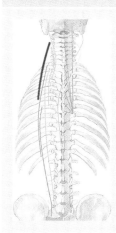

O: ribs 7–(6) 3 medial to the Angulus costae

I: Tuberculum posterius of the Proc. transversus of the cervical vertebrae C6–(C4) C3

F: unilaterally active:
- lateroflexion
bilaterally active:
- extension
- braces the spinal column

Trunk

a Sacrospinal system (continued)

M. longissimus thoracis
Rr. posteriores of the Nn. spinales

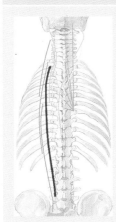

O: Procc. spinosi of the lumbar vertebrae, Facies dorsalis of the Os sacrum, frequently from the Proc. mamillaris of the lumbar vertebrae L2 and L1 as well as from the Proc. transversus of the thoracic vertebrae T12–T6

I: medial part: Proc. mamillaris of the lumbar vertebra L5,
Proc. accessorius of the lumbar vertebrae L4–L1,
Procc. transversi of the thoracic vertebrae;
lateral part: Proc. costalis of the lumbar vertebrae L4–L1,
deep lamina of the Fascia thoracolumbalis,
ribs 12–2 medial to the Angulus costae

F: unilaterally active:
• lateroflexion
bilaterally active:
• extension
• braces the spinal column

M. longissimus cervicis
Rr. posteriores of the Nn. spinales

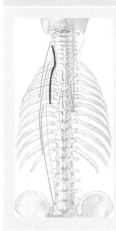

O: Proc. transversus of the thoracic T6–T1 and cervical vertebrae C7–C3

I: Tuberculum posterius of the Proc. transversus of the cervical vertebrae C5–C2

F: unilaterally active:
• lateroflexion
bilaterally active:
• extension
• braces the spinal column

M. longissimus capitis
Rr. posteriores of the Nn. spinales

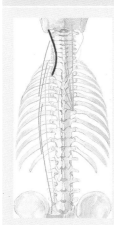

O: Proc. transversus of the thoracic to the cervical vertebrae T3–C3

I: posterior margin of the Proc. mastoideus

F: unilaterally active:
• lateroflexion
bilaterally active:
• extension
• braces the spinal column

b Intertransversal system

Mm. intertransversarii laterales lumborum (These are not autochthonous muscles in the true sense, but are instead of ventral origin.)
Rr. anteriores of the Nn. spinales

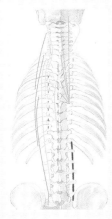

O: Tuberositas iliaca,
Proc. costalis and Proc. accessorius of the lumbar vertebrae L5–L1,
Proc. transversus of the thoracic vertebra C12

I: Proc. costalis of the lumbar vertebrae L5–L1, Tuberositas iliaca

F: unilaterally active:
• lateroflexion
bilaterally active:
• extension

Mm. intertransversarii mediales lumborum
Rr. posteriores of the Nn. spinales

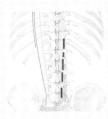

O: Proc. accessorius of the lumbar vertebrae L4–L1

I: Proc. accessorius and Proc. mamillaris of the lumbar vertebrae L5–L2

F: unilaterally active:
• lateroflexion
bilaterally active:
• extension

Mm. intertransversarii thoracis
Rr. posteriores of the Nn. spinales

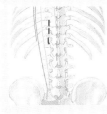

O: Proc. transversus of the thoracic vertebrae T12–T10

I: Proc. accessorius and Proc. mamillaris of the lumbar vertebra L1 up to the Proc. transversus of the thoracic vertebra T11

F: unilaterally active:
• lateroflexion
bilaterally active:
• extension

Mm. intertransversarii posteriores cervicis
Rr. posteriores of the Nn. spinales

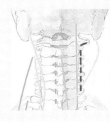

O: Tuberculum posterius of the Proc. transversus of the cervical vertebrae C4–C1

I: Tuberculum posterius of the Proc. transversus of the cervical vertebrae C5–C2

F: unilaterally active:
• lateroflexion
bilaterally active:
• extension

Mm. intertransversarii anteriores cervicis (These are not autochthonous muscles in the true sense, but are instead of ventral origin.)
Rr. anteriores of the Nn. spinales

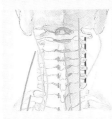

O: Tuberculum anterius of the Proc. transversus of the cervical vertebrae C6–C1

I: Tuberculum anterius of the Proc. transversus of the cervical vertebrae C7–C2

F: unilaterally active:
• lateroflexion
bilaterally active:
• extension

Trunk

c Spinotransversal system

M. splenius cervicis
Rr. posteriores of the Nn. cervicales

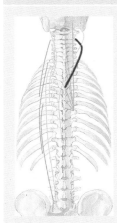

O: Proc. spinosus of the thoracic vertebrae T3–T6, Lig. supraspinale

I: Tuberculum posterius of the Proc. transversus of the cervical vertebrae C2–C1 (sometimes also C3)

F: unilaterally active:
- lateroflexion
- rotation of the cervical spine and of the head to the ipsilateral side

bilaterally active:
- extension of the cervical spine
- braces the cervical spine

M. splenius capitis
Rr. posteriores of the Nn. cervicales

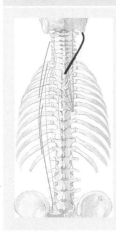

O: Proc. spinosus of the cervical vertebrae C3–C7, Lig. supraspinale, Lig. nuchae

I: Proc. mastoideus, (Linea nuchalis superior)

F: unilaterally active:
- lateroflexion,
- rotation of the cervical spine and of the head to the ipsilateral side

bilaterally active:
- extension of the cervical spine
- braces the cervical spine

d Mm. levatores costarum

(The 12 pairs of Mm. levatores costarum are back muscles which cannot uniformly be assigned to a specific group. They are innervated by the Rr. posteriores of the spinal nerves and additionally by small branches of the Rr. ventrales of the intercostal nerves. It is assumed that they have migrated from the transverse processes to the ribs. They are therefore partly categorised in the literature as secondary back muscles which have migrated. The Mm. levatores costarum longi each skip a rib, while the Mm. levatores costarum breves continue to the next caudal rib.)
Rr. posteriores of the N. cervicalis [C8] and of the Nn. thoracici [T1–T10]

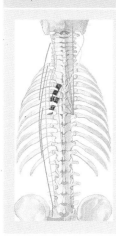

O: Proc. transversus of the thoracic to cervical vertebrae T11 to C7

I: ribs 12–1, each lateral of the Angulus costae

F: lift the ribs, lateroflexion and rotation of the spinal column

19.2 Medial tract

The medial tract of the autochthonous muscles of the back is located beneath the lateral tract in the cervical and lumbar regions. Hence, it is also referred to as the deep part of the autochthonous muscles of the back. The Mm. interspinales and the M. spinalis constitute the group of straight muscles. The Mm. rotatores, the Mm. multifidi and the M. semispinalis converge in an oblique craniomedial direction (transversospinal).

a Spinal system

Mm. interspinales lumborum
Rr. posteriores of the Nn. spinales

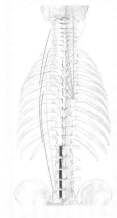

O: Proc. spinosus of the lumbar vertebrae L5–L1

I: superior rim of the Crista sacralis mediana, Proc. spinosus of the lumbar vertebrae L5–L2

F: segmental extension, stabilisation and fine-tuning of the motion segments

---

Mm. interspinales thoracis
Rr. posteriores of the Nn. spinales

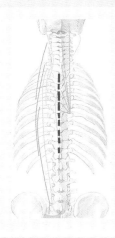

O: Proc. spinosus of the thoracic vertebrae (T12) T11–T2 (T1)

I: Proc. spinosus of the (L1 lumbar) thoracic vertebrae T12–T3 (T2)

F: segmental extension, stabilisation and fine-tuning of the motion segments

---

Mm. interspinales cervicis
Rr. posteriores of the Nn. spinales

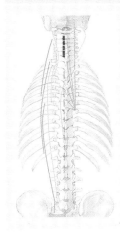

O: Proc. spinosus of the cervical vertebrae C7–C2

I: Proc. spinosus of the thoracic to cervical vertebrae T1–C3

F: segmental extension, stabilisation and fine-tuning of the motion segments

---

Trunk

a Spinal system (continued)

M. spinalis thoracis (At its origin and insertion, this muscle has close connections with the M. longissimus thoracis and the Mm. multifidi, respectively.)
Rr. posteriores of the Nn. spinales

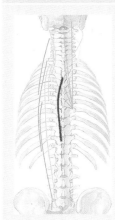

O: Proc. spinosus of the lumbar (L3) L2, L1 and thoracic vertebrae T12–T10

I: Proc. spinosus of the thoracic vertebrae (T10) T9–T2

F: unilaterally active:
- lateroflexion

bilaterally active:
- extension

M. spinalis cervicis
Rr. posteriores of the Nn. spinales

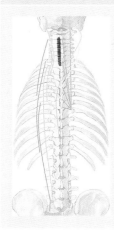

O: Proc. spinosus of the thoracic (T4) T3–T1 and cervical vertebrae C7–C6

I: Proc. spinosus of the cervical vertebrae (C6) C5–C2

F: unilaterally active:
- lateroflexion

bilaterally active:
- extension

M. spinalis capitis (inconstant muscle, closely connected to the M. semispinalis capitis via a shared attachment)
Rr. posteriores of the Nn. spinales

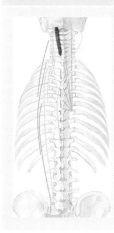

O: Proc. spinosus of the thoracic T3–T1 and cervical vertebrae C7–C6

I: Squama ossis occipitalis between Linea nuchalis suprema and Linea nuchalis superior close to the Protuberantia occipitalis externa

F: unilaterally active:
- lateroflexion

bilaterally active:
- extension

b Transversospinal system

Mm. rotatores (They are subdivided into the Mm. rotatores cervicis, Mm. rotatores thoracis and the inconstant Mm. rotatores lumborum. The Mm. rotatores breves run to the adjacent upper vertebra, whereas the Mm. rotatores longi skip one vertebra at a time.)
Rr. posteriores of the Nn. spinales

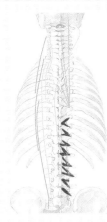

O: Procc. mamillares of the lumbar vertebrae, Procc. transversi of the thoracic vertebrae, Procc. articulares inferiores of the cervical vertebrae

I: base of the Proc. spinosus of the lumbar L3–L1, thoracic T12–T1, and cervical vertebrae C7–C2

F: unilaterally active:
- segmental lateroflexion
- rotation

bilaterally active:
- segmental extension
- stabilisation of the motion segments

Mm. multifidi (They are particularly strong in the lumbar region and skip two to four vertebrae at a time.)
Rr. posteriores of the Nn. spinales

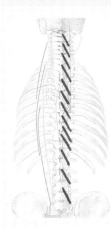

O: Facies dorsalis of the Os sacrum, Lig. sacroiliacum posterius, corsal part of the Crista iliaca, Procc. mamillares of the lumbar vertebrae, Procc. transversi of the thoracic vertebrae, Proc. articularis inferior of the cervical vertebrae C7–C4

I: Proc. spinosus of the lumbar L5–L1, thoracic T12–T1, and cervical vertebrae C7–C2

F: unilaterally active:
- segmental lateroflexion
- rotation

bilaterally active:
- segmental extension
- brace and stabilise the spinal column

M. semispinalis thoracis (Its muscle fibres skip five to seven vertebrae at a time.)
Rr. posteriores of the Nn. spinales

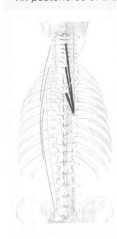

O: Proc. transversus of the thoracic vertebrae (T12) T11–T7 (T6)

I: Proc. spinosus of the thoracic to the cervical vertebrae (T4) T3–C6

F: unilaterally active:
- rotation of the spinal column and head to the contralateral side

bilaterally active:
- extension
- brace and stabilise the spinal column

b Transversospinal system (continued)

M. semispinalis cervicis
Rr. posteriores of the Nn. spinales

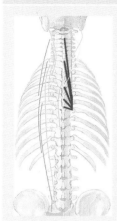

O: Proc. transversus of the thoracic to cervical vertebrae (T7) T6–C7

I: Proc. spinosus of the cervical vertebrae C6–C3

F: unilaterally active:
- rotation of the spinal column and head to the contralateral side
- side inclination

bilaterally active:
- extension
- brace and stabilise the thoracic and cervical parts of the spinal column

M. semispinalis capitis
Rr. posteriores of the Nn. spinales

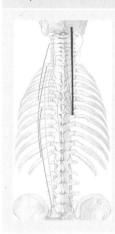

O: Proc. transversus of the thoracic to cervical vertebrae (T8) T7–C3

I: Squama ossis occipitalis between the Linea nuchalis suprema and Linea nuchalis superior, medial part

F: unilaterally active:
- rotation of the spinal column and head to the contralateral side
- side inclination

bilaterally active:
- extension
- brace and stabilise the thoracic and cervical parts of the spinal column

19.3 Autochthonous deep muscles of the neck

M. rectus capitis posterior major
N. suboccipitalis (dorsal branch of the N. cervicalis [C1])

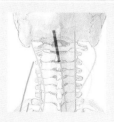

O: Proc. spinosus of the axis

I: middle third of the Linea nuchalis inferior

F: unilaterally active:
- rotates and inclines the head to the ipsilateral side

bilaterally active:
- involved in the fine-tuning of the position and kinematics of the head joints
- extension, fine-tuning of the position of the head in the atlanto-occipital joint

M. rectus capitis posterior minor
N. suboccipitalis (dorsal branch of the N. cervicalis [C1])

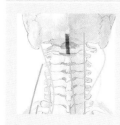

O: Tuberculum posterius of the Arcus posterior of the atlas

I: inferomedial to the Linea nuchalis inferior

F: unilaterally active:
- rotates and inclines the head to the ipsilateral side

bilaterally active:
- involved in the fine-tuning of the position and kinematics of the head joints
- extension, fine-tuning of the position of the head in the atlanto-occipital joint

19.3 Autochthonous deep muscles of the neck (continued)

M. obliquus capitis superior
N. suboccipitalis (dorsal branch of the N. cervicalis [C1])

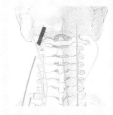

O: Proc. transversus of the atlas

I: lateral third of the Linea nuchalis inferior

F: unilaterally active:
- inclines the head to the ipsilateral side

bilaterally active:
- involved in the fine-tuning of the position and kinematics of the head joints
- extension

M. obliquus capitis inferior
N. suboccipitalis (dorsal branch of the N. cervicalis [C1])

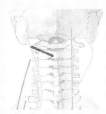

O: Proc. spinosus of the axis

I: Proc. transversus of the atlas

F: unilaterally active:
- rotates the head to the ipsilateral side

bilaterally active:
- involved in the fine-tuning of the position and kinematics of the head joints
- extension

20 Movements of the head joint and cervical spine

Movement	Muscles involved in the movement
C0–C1-joint	
Flexion	M. longus capitis, M. rectus capitis anterior
Extension	M. rectus capitis posterior, M semispinalis capitis, M. splenius capitis, M. obliquus capitis superior, M. sternocleidomastoideus, M. trapezius
Lateral flexion	M. rectus capitis lateralis, M. splenius capitis, M. semispinalis capitis, M. sternocleidomastoideus (of the same side), M. trapezius (of the same side)
C1–C2-joint	
Rotation – ipsilateral contraction	M. obliquus capitis superior, M. obliquus capitis inferior, M. rectus capitis posterior, M. splenius capitis, M. longissimus capitis
Rotation – contralateral contraction	M. sternocleidomastoideus, M. semispinalis capitis
C2–C7	
Flexion	M. sternocleidomastoideus, Mm. scaleni, M. longus capitis, M. rectus capitis anterior
Extension	M. splenius capitis, M. semispinalis capitis, M. semispinalis cervicis, M. splenius cervicis, M. semispinalis thoracis, M. rectus capitis posterior, M. obliquus capitis
Lateral flexion	Mm. scaleni, M. longus capitis, M. rectus capitis lateralis, M. longus colli, M. semispinalis capitis, M. semispinalis cervicis, M. semispinalis thoracis
Rotation	M. sternocleidomastoideus, M splenius capitis, M. longus capitis, M. longus colli, M. rectus capitis posterior, M. obliquus capitis, M. semispinalis thoracis, M. semispinalis capitis, M. semispinalis cervicis, M. splenius cervicis

21 Diaphragm

The diaphragm separates the thoracic cavity from the abdominal cavity. Its domes form the floor of the right and left pleural cavity, respectively. The Pars lumbalis delineates the retroperitoneal space dorsally and is part of the posterior abdominal wall.

21.1 Muscle

Diaphragma
N. phrenicus (Plexus cervicalis)

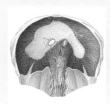

O: Pars sternalis: inner surface of the Proc. xiphoideus, rectus sheath and aponeurosis of the M. transversus abdominis
Pars costalis: inner surface of the Cartilago costalis of ribs 12–6
Pars lumbalis:
- Crus mediale: corpus of the fourth–first lumbar vertebra and the intervertebral discs (Lig. longitudinale anterius, Lig. arcuatum intermedium)
- Crus intermedium: lateral surface of the second lumbar vertebra
- Crus laterale: attaches with the Ligg. arcuata mediale (psoas arcade) and laterale (quadratus arcade) to the Proc. costalis of the first (second) lumbar vertebra, of the 12th rib

I: all parts unite in the Centrum tendineum

F: diaphragmatic (abdominal) breathing (inspiration), abdominal press

21.2 Passageways and weak spots in the diaphragm

Name	Position	Structures
Hiatus aorticus	Pars lumbalis, between the Crus dextrum, Crus sinistrum and spinal column	• Aorta • Ductus thoracicus
Hiatus oesophageus	Pars lumbalis (Pars medialis, left side)	• Oesophagus • Nn. vagi • N. phrenicus sinister: R. phrenicoabdominalis sinister
Foramen venae cavae	Centrum tendineum	• V. cava inferior • N. phrenicus dexter: R. phrenicoabdominalis dexter
Trigonum sternocostale [LARREY's triangle]	between the Pars sternalis and Pars costalis	A./V. epigastrica superior
Trigonum lumbocostale [BOCHDALEK's triangle]	between the Pars costalis and Pars lumbalis	
Not labeled	Pars lumbalis, (Pars medialis)	• N. splanchnicus major and minor • V. azygos • V. hemiazygos
Not labeled	Pars lumbalis, between the Pars medialis and Pars lateralis	Truncus sympathicus
Not labeled	Centrum tendineum	N. phrenicus sinister: R. phrenicoabdominalis sinister

22 Pelvic floor, perineal and sphincter muscles of the anus

The pelvic diaphragm is formed by the M. levator ani and the M. ischiococcygeus. Beneath it lie the perineal muscles.

22.1 Pelvic floor (Diaphragma pelvis)

M. levator ani (It consists of the M. pubococcygeus and the M. iliococcygeus. Beginning at the M. pubococcygeus, the M. puborectalis forms a loop around the rectum.)
Branches of the N. sacralis [S3 and S4], M. puborectalis through the N. pudendus

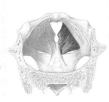

O: M. pubococcygeus: inner surface of the Os pubis close to the Symphysis pubica
M. iliococcygeus: Arcus tendineus musculi levatoris ani

I: Centrum tendineum perinei, Os coccygis, Os sacrum, loop formation with fibres of the opposite side behind the anus (M. puborectalis)

F: stabilises the pelvic organs, thereby facilitating urinary and faecal continence; encompasses the rectum from behind, hence distal rectal occlusion (M. puborectalis)

M. ischiococcygeus
Branches of the N. sacralis [S3 and S4]

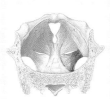

O: Spina ischiadica, Lig. sacrospinale

I: Os sacrum, Os coccygis

F: similar to M. levator ani

22.2 Perineal muscles

M. transversus perinei profundus
N. pudendus (Plexus sacralis)

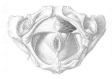

O: Ramus inferior ossis pubis

I: Centrum tendineum perinei

F: secures the levator gap

M. sphincter urethrae externus (part of the M. transversus perinei profundus)
N. pudendus (Plexus sacralis)

O: circular muscle, muscle fibres from the M. transversus perinei profundus

I: connective tissue surrounding the urethra (Pars membranacea), vaginal wall (M. sphincter urethrovaginalis)

F: occlusion of the urethra

M. transversus perinei superficialis (inconstant muscle)
N. pudendus (Plexus sacralis)

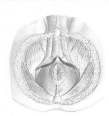

O: Ramus ossis ischii

I: Centrum tendineum perinei

F: supports the M. transversus perinei profundus

Trunk

22.2 Perineal muscles (continued)

M. ischiocavernosus
N. pudendus (Plexus sacralis)

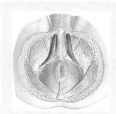

O: Ramus ossis ischii

I: Crus penis/clitoridis

F: stabilises the cavernous bodies of the penis/clitoris, ejaculation

M. bulbospongiosus (surrounds the Bulbus penis in men and the Bulbus vestibuli in women)
N. pudendus (Plexus sacralis)

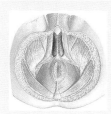

O: Centrum tendineum perinei, in men also at the Raphe penis

I: encompasses the Bulbus penis/ Bulbus vestibuli

F: stabilises the cavernous bodies of the penis/clitoris, ejaculation

22.3 Sphincter muscles of the anus

M. sphincter ani externus
N. pudendus (Plexus sacralis)

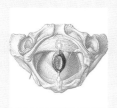

O: Pars subcutanea: dermis and subcutis around the anus
Pars superficialis and Pars profunda: Centrum tendineum perinei

I: dermis and subcutis around the anus, Lig. anococcygeum

F: occlusion of the anus

Upper limb

Plexus brachialis
M. pectoralis minor
M. subclavius
M. serratus anterior
M. pectoralis major
M. deltoideus
M. supraspinatus
M. trapezius
M. levator scapulae
M. rhomboideus minor
M. rhomboideus major
M. infraspinatus
M. teres minor
M. teres major
M. subscapularis
M. latissimus dorsi
M. biceps brachii
M. coracobrachialis
M. brachialis
M. triceps brachii
M. anconeus
M. pronator teres
M. flexor carpi radialis
M. palmaris longus
M. flexor digitorum superficialis
M. flexor carpi ulnaris

M. flexor digitorum profundus
M. flexor pollicis longus
M. pronator quadratus
M. brachioradialis
M. extensor carpi radialis longus
M. extensor carpi radialis brevis
M. extensor digitorum
M. extensor digiti minimi
M. extensor carpi ulnaris
M. supinator
M. abductor pollicis longus
M. extensor pollicis brevis
M. extensor pollicis longus
M. extensor indicis
M. abductor pollicis brevis
M. flexor pollicis brevis
M. opponens pollicis
M. adductor pollicis
Mm. lumbricales I–IV
Mm. interossei palmares I–III
Mm. interossei dorsales I–IV
M. palmaris brevis
M. abductor digiti minimi
M. flexor digiti minimi brevis
M. opponens digiti minimi

Upper limb

23 Joints of the upper limb, Articulationes membri superioris

23.1 Joints of the shoulder girdle, Articulationes cinguli pectoralis

Name of joint	Type of joint	Types of movements
Medial clavicular joint Articulatio sternoclavicularis	uneven articular surfaces, Articulatio irregularis, functionally: spheroidal joint, (characteristic: Discus articularis)	• rotation around the sagittal axis (when lifting the shoulder) • rotation around the longitudinal axis of the arm (during anteversion and retroversion of the shoulder) • rotation around the longitudinal axis of the clavicle (when swinging the arm)
Lateral clavicular joint Articulatio acromioclavicularis	planar joint, Articulatio plana, functionally: spheroidal joint, (characteristic: variable, mostly incomplete Discus articularis)	• rotation around a sagittal axis (when lifting the shoulder) • rotation around a transverse axis (when swinging the arm) • rotation around a longitudinal axis (during anteversion and retroversion of the shoulder)

23.2 Joints of the free upper limb, Articulationes membri superioris liberi

Joint name		Joint type	Types of movements
Shoulder joint Articulatio humeri		ball joint, Articulatio spheroidea	• leaning forward, anteversion (bending, flexion) • leaning backward, retroversion (stretching, extension) • lateral raises, abduction • towards the centre of the body, adduction • internal rotation • external rotation • (arm circling, circumduction: combined movement of anteversion, abduction, retroversion, adduction)
Elbow joint Articulatio cubiti	Humeroulnar joint, Articulatio humeroulnaris	hinge joint, ginglymus	• bending, flexion • stretching, extension
	Humeroradial joint, Articulatio humeroradialis	ball joint, Articulatio spheroidea (functionally restricted: no abduction)	• bending, flexion • stretching, extension • arm circling, rotation
	Proximal radioulnar joint, Articulatio radioulnaris proximalis	pivot joint, Articulatio conoidea	turning movements of the hand, pronation and supination
Distal radioulnar joint Articulatio radioulnaris distalis		pivot joint, Articulatio trochoidea	
Hand joints	Proximal hand joint, Articulatio radiocarpalis	ellipsoidal joint, Articulatio ellipsoidea	• sideways movements of the hand, abduction toward ulnar or radial • bending, palmar flexion • stretching, dorsal extension
	Distal hand joint, Articulatio mediocarpalis	interlocking hinge joint, ginglymus	
Carpometacarpal joint of the thumb Articulatio carpometacarpalis pollicis		saddle joint, Articulatio sellaris	• splaying out, abduction • closing, adduction • opposing, opposition • repositioning, reposition
Carpometacarpal joints II–V Articulationes carpometacarpales II–V		saddle joint, Articulatio sellaris	differ greatly
Metacarpophalangeal joints Articulationes metacarpophalangeae		ball joints, Articulationes spheroideae (functionally restricted)	• bending, flexion • stretching, extension • splaying out, abduction* • closing, adduction* (* related to the middle finger)
Metacarpophalangeal joints Articulationes metacarpophalangeae		hinge joints, ginglymi	• bending, flexion • stretching, extension

23.3 Planes and axes of movement of joints of the upper limb

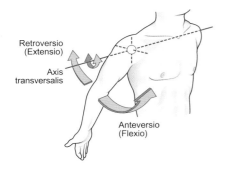

Fig. 1 Shoulder joint;
movement in the sagittal plane. [S700-L126]

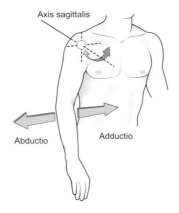

Fig. 2 Shoulder joint;
movement in the frontal plane.
[S700-L126]

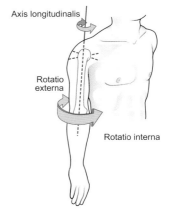

Fig. 3 Shoulder joint;
movement in the transverse plane.
[S700-L126]

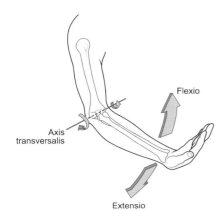

Fig. 4 Elbow joint;
movement in the sagittal plane. [S700-L126]

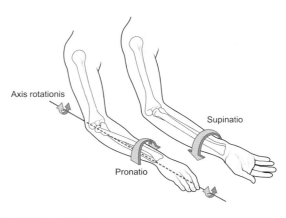

Fig. 5 Elbow joint;
rotational movement of the hand. [S700-L126]

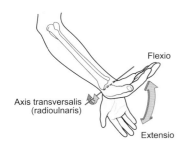

Fig. 6 Carpal joint;
movement in the sagittal plane (planar
movements). [S700-L126]

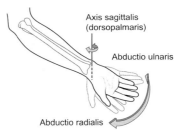

Fig. 7 Carpal joint;
movement in the frontal plane (marginal
movements). [S700-L126]

Palmar flexion and dorsiflexion in the carpal joint are also known as flexion and extension, respectively.

24 Branches and innervation areas of the Plexus brachialis

The **brachial plexus (Plexus brachialis)** is composed of the Rr. anteriores of the spinal nerves from the spinal cord segments **C5–T1** (variably also from C3–C4 and T2). It is important to note that not all spinal cord segments which send fibres into individual nerves of the brachial plexus take part equally in the innervation of all muscles. As certain segments predominate in some muscles, as shown in → Tab. 25, these can be used as key muscles in clinical diagnostics.

Branch	Motor	Sensory
N. dorsalis scapulae C3–C5	M. levator scapulae, Mm. rhomboidei	
N. suprascapularis C4–C6	M. supraspinatus, M. infraspinatus	
Nn. subscapulares C5–C7	M. subscapularis, (M. teres major)	
N. subclavius C5, C6	M. subclavius	
N. thoracicus longus C5–C7	M. serratus anterior	
Nn. pectorales C5–T1	M. pectoralis major, M. pectoralis minor	
N. thoracodorsalis C6–C8	M. latissimus dorsi, M. teres major	
Rr. musculares	M. longus colli, M. longus capitis	
N. musculocutaneus C5–C7	M. coracobrachialis, M. biceps brachii, M. brachialis	skin of the radial palmar side of the forearm
N. medianus C6–T1	M. pronator teres, M. flexor carpi radialis, M. palmaris longus, M. flexor digitorum superficialis, M. flexor pollicis longus, M. flexor digitorum profundus (radial part), M. pronator quadratus, M. flexor pollicis brevis (Caput superficiale), M. opponens pollicis, Mm. lumbricales I, II	skin of the radial part of the palm (3½ fingers), skin of the dorsal distal phalanges (3½ fingers)
N. ulnaris C8–T1	M. flexor carpi ulnaris, M. flexor digitorum profundus (ulnar part), M. palmaris brevis, M. flexor digiti minimi, M. opponens digiti minimi, M. abductor digiti minimi, M. flexor pollicis brevis (Caput profundum), M. adductor pollicis, Mm. lumbricales III, IV, Mm. interossei	skin of the ulnar side of the hand (palmar: 1½ fingers, dorsal: 2½ fingers), skin of the dorsal distal phalanges (1½ fingers)
N. cutaneus brachii medialis C8–T1		skin of the medial palmar side of the upper arm
N. cutaneus antebrachii medialis C8–T1		skin of the ulnar palmar side of the forearm
N. axillaris C5–C6	M. deltoideus, M. teres minor	skin of the shoulder
N. radialis C5–T1	M. triceps brachii, M. anconeus, M. brachioradialis, M. extensor carpi radialis longus, M. extensor carpi radialis brevis, M. supinator, M. extensor digitorum, M. extensor pollicis longus, M. abductor pollicis longus, M. extensor pollicis brevis, M. extensor indicis, M. extensor carpi ulnaris	skin of the dorsal side of the upper arm, forearm, and hand (2½ radial fingers, with the exception of the distal phalanges)

25 Segmental innervation of muscles of the upper limb, diagnostically important key muscles

The muscles printed in bold are used clinically as key muscles for a specific spinal cord segment.

Segmental innervation of muscles of the upper limb, diagnostically important key muscles

M. supraspinatus	C4–C5	M. abductor pollicis longus	C6–C8
M. teres minor	C4–C5	M. extensor pollicis brevis	C7–T1
M. deltoideus: C5	C5–C6	M. extensor pollicis longus	C6–C8
M. infraspinatus	C4–C6	M. extensor digitorum	C6–C8
M. subscapularis	C5–C6	M. extensor indicis	C6–C8
M. teres major	C5–C7	M. extensor carpi ulnaris	C6–C8
M. biceps brachii: C6	C5–C6	M. extensor digiti minimi	C6–C8
M. brachialis	C5–C6	M. flexor digitorum superficialis	C7–T1
M. coracobrachialis	C5–C7	M. flexor digitorum profundus	C7–T1
M. triceps brachii: C7	C6–C8	M. flexor carpi ulnaris	C7–T1
M. brachioradialis	C5–C6	M. abductor pollicis brevis	C7–T1
M. extensor carpi radialis longus	C5–C7	M. flexor pollicis brevis	C7–T1
M. extensor carpi radialis brevis	C5–C7	M. opponens pollicis	C6–C7
M. supinator	C5–C6	M. flexor digiti minimi	C7–T1
M. pronator teres	C6–C7	M. adductor pollicis	C8–T1
M. flexor carpi radialis	C6–C7	**M. abductor digiti minimi: C8**	C8–T1
M. flexor pollicis longus	C6–C8	**Mm. interossei: C8**	C8–T1

26 Ventral muscles of the shoulder girdle

The shoulder muscles are composed of two groups. The **muscles of the shoulder girdle** insert at the scapula or the clavicle and primarily move the shoulder girdle, and thereby only indirectly the arm. The **muscles of the shoulder** insert at the humerus and move it directly. The M. serratus anterior, M. pectoralis minor and M. subclavius represent the ventral muscles of the shoulder girdle.

M. pectoralis minor
Nn. pectorales medialis et lateralis (Plexus brachialis, Pars infraclavicularis)

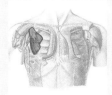

O: ribs (2) 3–5 close to the bone-cartilage junction

I: tip of the Proc. coracoideus

F: shoulder girdle:
- lowering

thorax:
- elevating the upper ribs
- (inspiration: auxiliary breathing muscle)

M. subclavius
N. subclavius (Plexus brachialis, Pars supraclavicularis)

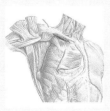

O: bone-cartilage junction of rib 1

I: lateral third of the clavicle

F: shoulder girdle:
- stabilises the sternoclavicular joint
- protects the Vasa subclavia

The fascia of the M. subclavius and the adventitia of the V. subclavia adhere tightly and this keeps the venous lumen open.

M. serratus anterior (A scapula alata is caused by the paralysis of the M. serratus anterior or the M. rhomboideus.)
N. thoracicus longus (Plexus brachialis, Pars supraclavicularis)

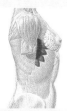

O: ribs 1–9

I: Pars superior: Angulus superior
Pars divergens: Margo medialis
Pars convergens: Angulus inferior

F: shoulder girdle:
- pulls the scapula ventrolaterally, presses the scapula against the thorax along with the Mm. rhomboidei
- **Pars superior:** elevates the scapula
- **Pars divergens:** lowers the scapula
- **Pars convergens:** lowers the scapula and, along with the M. trapezius, rotates its lower angle outwards to elevate the arm above the horizontal axis

thorax:
- elevates the ribs when the scapula is in a fixed position (inspiration)

Upper limb

27 Ventral muscles of the shoulder

The M. pectoralis major is the only ventral shoulder muscle and is responsible for the surface of the ventral upper chest wall.

M. pectoralis major (The muscle fibres converge laterally to form a broad flat tendon in a pocket-shape which is open at the top.)
Nn. pectorales medialis et lateralis (Plexus brachialis, Pars infraclavicularis)

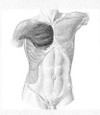

O: Pars clavicularis: sternal half of the clavicle
Pars sternocostalis: Manubrium and Corpus sterni, Cartilago costalis of ribs 2–7
Pars abdominalis: anterior lamina of the rectus sheath

I: Crista tuberculi majoris of the humerus

F: shoulder joint:
- adduction (most important muscle)
- medial rotation
- anteversion (most important muscle)
- retroversion from an anteverted position

thorax:
- elevates the sternum and upper ribs when the shoulder girdle is in a fixed position
- (inspiration: auxiliary breathing muscle)

28 Lateral muscles of the shoulder

The M. deltoideus distinctively shapes the surface of the shoulder. Beneath it and separated by the Bursa subdeltoidea lies the tendon of the M. supraspinatus.

M. deltoideus
N. axillaris (Plexus brachialis, Pars infraclavicularis)

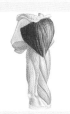

O: Pars clavicularis: acromial third of the clavicle
Pars acromialis: Acromion
Pars spinalis: Spina scapulae

I: Tuberositas deltoidea

F: shoulder joint:
- abduction (most important muscle)

Pars clavicularis:
- adduction (increasingly abducted from approx. 60° onwards),
- medial rotation
- anteversion

Pars acromialis:
- abduction up to the horizontal plane

Pars spinalis:
- adduction (increasingly abducted from approx. 60° onwards),
- lateral rotation
- retroversion

M. supraspinatus
N. suprascapularis (Plexus brachialis, Pars supraclavicularis)

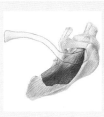

O: Fossa supraspinata, Fascia supraspinata

I: upper facet of the Tuberculum majus, joint capsule

F: shoulder joint:
- abduction up to the horizontal plane
- small degree of lateral rotation
- reinforcement of the joint capsule **(rotator cuff)**

29 Dorsal muscles of the shoulder girdle

The dorsal muscles of this group, M. trapezius, M. levator scapulae, M. rhomboideus major and M. rhomboideus minor, are considered as superficial muscles of the back due to their location. Their origin and innervation identifies them as muscles of the back that have migrated into the shoulder region.

M. trapezius
N. accessorius [XI] and branches of the Plexus cervicalis

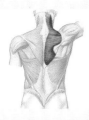

O: Pars descendens: Os occipitale between the Linea nuchalis suprema and Linea nuchalis superior
Pars transversa: Procc. spinosi of the cervical and thoracic vertebrae
Pars ascendens: Procc. spinosi of the thoracic vertebrae

I: Pars descendens: acromial third of the clavicle
Pars transversa: Acromion
Pars ascendens: Spina scapulae

F: Pars descendens:
- prevents lowering of the shoulder girdle and arm (e. g. carrying a suitcase)
- elevates the scapula and rotates its lower tip (Angulus inferior) laterally to allow the elevation of the arm above the horizontal plane, along with the M. serratus anterior
- rotates the head to the contralateral side when the shoulder is in a fixed position
- extends the cervical spine with bilateral innervation

Pars transversa:
- pulls the scapula downwards

Pars ascendens:
- lowers the scapula and rotates it downwards

M. levator scapulae
Direct branches of the Plexus cervicalis and N. dorsalis scapulae (Plexus brachialis, Pars supraclavicularis)

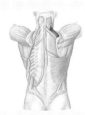

O: Tubercula posteriora of the Procc. transversi of the cervical vertebrae C1–C4

I: Angulus superior of the scapula

F: shoulder girdle:
- elevates the scapula

M. rhomboideus minor
N. dorsalis scapulae (Plexus brachialis, Pars supraclavicularis)

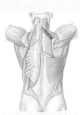

O: Proc. spinosus of the cervical vertebrae C6 and C7

I: Margo medialis of the scapula, cranial to the Spina scapulae

F: pulls the scapula medially and cranially, fixes the scapula to the torso, along with the M. serratus anterior

M. rhomboideus major
N. dorsalis scapulae (Plexus brachialis, Pars supraclavicularis)

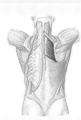

O: Proc. spinosus of the upper four thoracic vertebrae

I: Margo medialis of the scapula, caudal to the Spina scapulae

F: pulls the scapula medially and cranially, fixes the scapula to the torso along with the M. serratus anterior

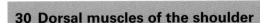

Upper limb

30 Dorsal muscles of the shoulder

The M. infraspinatus is located furthest cranially. Following caudally are the M. teres minor and the M. teres major. The M. subscapularis is the only muscle of this group located on the ventral side of the scapula. The M. latissimus dorsi covers a large area of the lower segments of the autochthonous muscles of the back.

M. infraspinatus
N. suprascapularis (Plexus brachialis, Pars supraclavicularis)

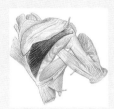

O: Fossa infraspinata, Fascia infraspinata

I: middle facet of the Tuberculum majus, joint capsule

F: shoulder joint:
- lateral rotation (most important muscle)
- reinforcement of the joint capsule **(rotator cuff)**

M. teres minor
N. axillaris (Plexus brachialis, Pars infraclavicularis)

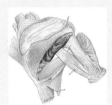

O: middle third of the Margo lateralis

I: lower facet of the Tuberculum majus, joint capsule

F: shoulder joint:
- lateral rotation
- adduction
- reinforcement of the joint capsule **(rotator cuff)**

M. teres major
N. thoracodorsalis (Plexus brachialis, Pars infraclavicularis)

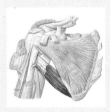

O: Angulus inferior

I: Crista tuberculi minoris medial to the M. latissimus dorsi

F: shoulder joint:
- medial rotation
- adduction
- retroversion

M. subscapularis (Beneath the muscle and adjacent to the insertion site lies the Bursa subtendinea musculi subscapularis.)
Nn. subscapulares (Plexus brachialis, Pars infraclavicularis)

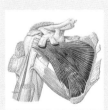

O: Fossa subscapularis

I: Tuberculum minus, joint capsule

F: shoulder joint:
- medial rotation (most important muscle)
- reinforcement of the joint capsule **(rotator cuff)**

M. latissimus dorsi
N. thoracodorsalis (Plexus brachialis, Pars infraclavicularis)

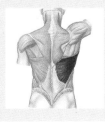

O: Proc. spinosus of the six lower thoracic vertebrae and the lumbar vertebrae, Fascia thoracolumbalis, Facies dorsalis of the Os sacrum, Labium externum of the Crista iliaca, ribs 9–12, frequently Angulus inferior of the scapula

I: Crista tuberculi minoris

F: shoulder joint:
- adduction
- medial rotation
- retroversion (most important muscle)

31 Ventral muscles of the upper arm

The M. biceps brachii shapes the surface of the ventral side of the upper arm. The M. coracobrachialis is in close proximity to its Caput breve. The M. brachialis is located in the deepest layer.

M. biceps brachii (The tendon of its Caput longum passes freely through the shoulder joint.)
N. musculocutaneus (Plexus brachialis, Pars infraclavicularis)

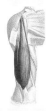

O: Caput longum: Tuberculum supraglenoidale
Caput breve: tip of the Proc. coracoideus

I: Tuberositas radii, via the Aponeurosis musculi bicipitis brachii at the Fascia antebrachii

F: shoulder joint:
- **Caput longum:** abduction, anteversion, medial rotation
- **Caput breve:** adduction, anteversion, medial rotation

elbow joint:
- flexion (most important muscle)
- supination (most important muscle with flexed elbow)

M. coracobrachialis (normally pierced by the N. musculocutaneus)
N. musculocutaneus (Plexus brachialis, Pars infraclavicularis)

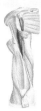

O: Proc. coracoideus

I: medially in the middle of the humerus

F: shoulder joint:
- medial rotation
- adduction
- anteversion

M. brachialis
N. musculocutaneus (Plexus brachialis, Pars infraclavicularis)

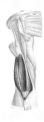

O: Facies anterior of the humerus (lower half)

I: Tuberositas ulnae

F: elbow joint:
- flexion
- tenses the joint capsule

32 Dorsal muscles of the upper arm

The three heads of the M. triceps brachii constitute the muscles at the dorsal side of the upper arm. Further distally, the M. anconeus is located further distally on the ulnar side at the transition to the forearm, and could be considered as the fourth head of the triceps muscle.

M. triceps brachii
N. radialis (Plexus brachialis, Pars infraclavicularis)

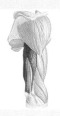

O: Caput longum: Tuberculum infraglenoidale
Caput mediale: Facies posterior of the humerus, medial and distal of the Sulcus nervi radialis
Caput laterale: Facies posterior of the humerus, lateral and proximal of the Sulcus nervi radialis

I: Olecranon

F: shoulder joint:
- **Caput longum:** adduction, retroversion

elbow joint:
- extension (most important muscle)

M. anconeus (located adjacent to the lateral part of the Caput mediale of the M. triceps brachii)
N. radialis (Plexus brachialis, Pars infraclavicularis)

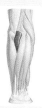

O: Epicondylus lateralis humeri

I: Facies posterior of the ulna, olecranon

F: elbow joint:
- extension

33 Ventral superficial muscles of the forearm

The M. pronator teres, M. flexor carpi radialis, M. palmaris longus and the M. flexor carpi ulnaris form the superficial layer. The M. flexor digitorum superficialis constitutes the middle layer.

M. pronator teres
N. medianus (Plexus brachialis, Pars infraclavicularis)

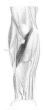

O: Caput humerale: Epicondylus medialis of the humerus
Caput ulnare: Proc. coronoideus

I: middle third of the Facies lateralis of the radius (Tuberositas pronatoria)

F: elbow joint:
- pronation (most important muscle)
- flexion

M. flexor carpi radialis
N. medianus (Plexus brachialis, Pars infraclavicularis)

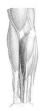

O: Epicondylus medialis of the humerus, Fascia antebrachii

I: palmar area of the base of the Os metacarpi II

F: elbow joint:
- flexion
- pronation
carpal joint: ·
- palmar flexion
- radial abduction

M. palmaris longus (inconstant muscle)
N. medianus (Plexus brachialis, Pars infraclavicularis)

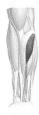

O: Epicondylus medialis of the humerus

I: Aponeurosis palmaris

F: elbow joint:
- flexion
carpal joint:
- palmar flexion
- tensing the palmar aponeurosis

M. flexor digitorum superficialis (Shortly before the tendons of this muscle reach their insertion sites, they are pierced by the tendons of the M. flexor digitorum profundus.)
N. medianus (Plexus brachialis, Pars infraclavicularis)

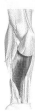

O: Caput humeroulnare: Epicondylus medialis of the humerus, Proc. coronoideus
Caput radiale: Facies anterior of the radius

I: with four long tendons at the base of the Phalanx media of the second to fifth fingers

F: elbow joint:
- flexion
carpal joint:
- palmar flexion
finger joints (II–V):
- flexion (most important flexor of the proximal interphalangeal joints)

M. flexor carpi ulnaris
N. ulnaris (Plexus brachialis, Pars infraclavicularis)

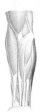

O: Caput humerale: Epicondylus medialis of the humerus
Caput ulnare: Olecranon, proximal at the Margo posterior of the ulna

I: via the Os pisiforme and the Ligg. pisometacarpale and pisohamatum at the base of the Os metacarpi V and the Os hamatum

F: elbow joint:
- flexion
carpal joint:
- palmar flexion
- ulnar abduction

34 Ventral deep muscles of the forearm

Located medially in the deep muscular layer is the M. flexor digitorum profundus and lateral thereof the M. flexor pollicis longus. The M. pronator quadratus covers the distal quarter of the forearm and represents the deepest layer.

M. flexor digitorum profundus
Ulnar part: N. ulnaris; radial part: N. interosseus antebrachii anterior from the N. medianus (Plexus brachialis, Pars infraclavicularis)

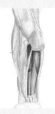

O: Facies anterior of the ulna, Membrana interossea

I: distal phalanges of the second to fifth fingers

F: carpal joint:
- palmar flexion

finger joints (II-V):
- flexion (most important flexor of the distal interphalangeal joints)

M. flexor pollicis longus
N. interosseus antebrachii anterior from the N. medianus (Plexus brachialis, Pars infraclavicularis)

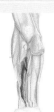

O: Facies anterior of the radius

I: distal phalanx of the thumb

F: carpal joint:
- palmar flexion

carpometacarpal joint:
- flexion
- opposition

interphalangeal joint:
- flexion

M. pronator quadratus
N. interosseus antebrachii anterior (N. medianus, Plexus brachialis, Pars infraclavicularis)

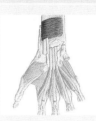

O: distal at the Facies anterior of the ulna

I: Facies anterior of the radius

F: radioulnar joints:
- pronation

35 Lateral (radial) muscles of the forearm

The group of radial muscles of the forearm consists of the M. brachioradialis, M. extensor carpi radialis longus and M. extensor carpi radialis brevis (from proximal to distal).

M. brachioradialis
N. radialis (Plexus brachialis, Pars infraclavicularis)

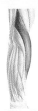

O: Margo lateralis of the humerus

I: proximal of the Proc. styloideus of the radius

F: elbow joint:
- flexion (because of the large virtual lever arm, this is particularly effective from a mid-flexed position)
- pronation or supination (facilitated pronation from the contralateral end-of-range positions)

M. extensor carpi radialis longus
N. radialis (Plexus brachialis, Pars infraclavicularis)

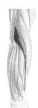

O: Crista supraepicondylaris lateralis up to the Epicondylus lateralis

I: dorsal area of the Os metacarpi II

F: elbow joint:
- flexion
- small degree of pronation (facilitated from the opposite end-of-range position)

carpal joint:
- dorsiflexion
- radial abduction

M. extensor carpi radialis brevis
N. radialis (Plexus brachialis, Pars infraclavicularis)

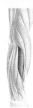

O: Epicondylus lateralis of the humerus

I: dorsal area of the Os metacarpi III

F: elbow joint:
- flexion
- small degree of pronation (facilitated from the opposite end-of-range position)

carpal joint:
- dorsiflexion
- radial abduction

Upper limb

36 Dorsal superficial muscles of the forearm

The group of dorsal superficial muscles of the forearm is composed of the M. extensor digitorum, the M. extensor digiti minimi and the M. extensor carpi ulnaris (from radial to ulnar).

M. extensor digitorum
R. profundus of the N. radialis (Plexus brachialis, Pars infraclavicularis)

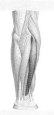

O: Epicondylus lateralis of the humerus, Fascia antebrachii

I: dorsal aponeurosis of the second to fifth fingers

F: elbow joint:
• extension
carpal joint:
• dorsiflexion
finger joints (II–V):
• extension (most important extensor of the metacarpophalangeal and proximal interphalangeal joints)

M. extensor digiti minimi
R. profundus of the N. radialis (Plexus brachialis, Pars infraclavicularis)

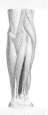

O: Epicondylus lateralis of the humerus, Fascia antebrachii

I: so-called dorsal aponeurosis of the fifth finger

F: elbow joint:
• extension
carpal joint:
• dorsiflexion
finger joint (V):
• extension (most important extensor of the metacarpophalangeal and proximal interphalangeal joints)

M. extensor carpi ulnaris
R. profundus of the N. radialis (Plexus brachialis, Pars infraclavicularis)

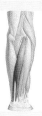

O: Caput humerale: Epicondylus lateralis of the humerus
Caput ulnare: Olecranon, Facies posterior of the ulna, Fascia antebrachii

I: dorsal area of the Os metacarpi V

F: elbow joint:
• extension
carpal joint:
• dorsiflexion
• ulnar abduction

37 Dorsal deep muscles of the forearm

The M. supinator wraps laterally around the upper (proximal) third of the radius. Following distally (from radial to ulnar) are the M. abductor pollicis longus, M. extensor pollicis brevis, M. extensor pollicis longus and the M. extensor indicis.

M. supinator (The R. profundus of the N. radialis pierces this muscle in the longitudinal direction of the forearm. The entrance point of the nerve into the supinator canal is marked by a small tendinous arch [FROHSE-FRÄNKEL's arcade].)
R. profundus of the N. radialis (Plexus brachialis, Pars infraclavicularis)

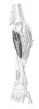

O: Epicondylus lateralis humeri, Crista musculi supinatoris of the ulna, Ligg. collaterale radiale and anulare radii

I: Facies anterior of the radius (proximal third)

F: radioulnar joints:
- supination (most important muscle with extended elbow)

M. abductor pollicis longus
R. profundus of the N. radialis (Plexus brachialis, Pars infraclavicularis)

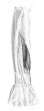

O: Facies posterior of ulna and radius, Membrana interossea

I: base of the Os metacarpi I

F: carpal joint:
- dorsiflexion

carpometacarpal joint:
- abduction

M. extensor pollicis brevis
R. profundus of the N. radialis (Plexus brachialis, Pars infraclavicularis)

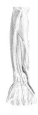

O: Facies posterior of ulna and radius, Membrana interossea

I: proximal phalanx of the thumb

F: carpal joint:
- dorsiflexion

carpometacarpal joint:
- abduction
- reposition

metacarpophalangeal joint:
- extension

M. extensor pollicis longus
R. profundus of the N. radialis (Plexus brachialis, Pars infraclavicularis)

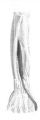

O: distal half of the Facies posterior of the ulna and radius, Membrana interossea

I: distal phalanx of the thumb

F: carpal joint:
- dorsiflexion

carpometacarpal joint:
- extension
- reposition

metacarpophalangeal joint:
- extension

M. extensor indicis
R. profundus of the N. radialis (Plexus brachialis, Pars infraclavicularis)

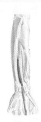

O: distal half of the Facies posterior of the ulna, Membrana interossea

I: dorsal aponeurosis of the index finger

F: carpal joint:
- dorsiflexion

finger joints (II):
- extension
- adduction

38 Thenar muscles

The thenar eminence is composed of the M. abductor pollicis brevis, M. flexor pollicis brevis and M. adductor pollicis (from radial to ulnar). The M. opponens pollicis lies beneath the M. abductor pollicis brevis.

M. abductor pollicis brevis
N. medianus (Plexus brachialis, Pars infraclavicularis)

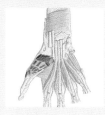

O: Retinaculum musculorum flexorum, Eminentia carpi radialis

I: radial sesamoid bone of the metacarpophalangeal joint, proximal phalanx of the thumb

F: carpometacarpal joint:
- abduction
- opposition

metacarpophalangeal joint:
- flexion

M. flexor pollicis brevis
Caput superficiale: N. medianus; Caput profundum: R. profundus of the N. ulnaris (Plexus brachialis, Pars infraclavicularis)

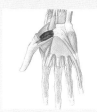

O: Caput superficiale: Retinaculum musculorum flexorum
Caput profundum: Os capitatum, Os trapezium

I: radial sesamoid bone of the metacarpophalangeal joint, proximal phalanx of the thumb

F: carpometacarpal joint:
- opposition
- adduction

metacarpophalangeal joint:
- flexion

M. opponens pollicis
N. medianus and N. ulnaris (Plexus brachialis, Pars infraclavicularis)

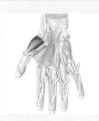

O: Retinaculum musculorum flexorum, Eminentia carpi radialis

I: Os metacarpi I

F: carpometacarpal joint:
- opposition

M. adductor pollicis
R. profundus of the N. ulnaris (Plexus brachialis, Pars infraclavicularis)

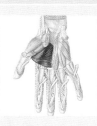

O: Caput obliquum: Os hamatum, Ossa metacarpi 2–4
Caput transversum: Os metacarpi 3

I: ulnar sesamoid bone of the metacarpophalangeal joint, proximal phalanx of the thumb

F: carpometacarpal joint:
- adduction
- opposition

metacarpophalangeal joint:
- flexion

39 Palmar muscles

The Mm. lumbricales originate from the tendons of the M. flexor digitorum profundus. The Mm. interossei palmares and the Mm. interossei dorsales fill the spaces between the Ossa metacarpi.

Mm. lumbricales I–IV
N. medianus (I, II); N. ulnaris (III, IV) (Plexus brachialis, Pars infraclavicularis)

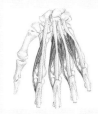

O: tendons II–IV of the M. flexor digitorum profundus (I + II from the radial side; III + IV from the sides facing each other, two-headed)

I: projecting radially into the dorsal aponeurosis (lateral tract) of the second to fifth fingers

F: metacarpophalangeal joints (II–V):
• flexion
interphalangeal joints (II–V):
• extension (most important extensors of the distal interphalangeal joints)

Mm. interossei palmares I–III
R. profundus, N. ulnaris (Plexus brachialis, Pars infraclavicularis)

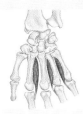

O: ulnar side of the Os metacarpi II, radial side of the Ossa metacarpi IV and V

I: proximal phalanx and dorsal aponeurosis (lateral tract) of the second, fourth and fifth fingers

F: metacarpophalangeal joints (II, IV, V):
• flexion (most important flexors!)
• adduction (with reference to the axis of the middle finger)
interphalangeal joints (II, IV, V):
• extension

Mm. interossei dorsales I–IV (two-headed)
R. profundus, N. ulnaris (Plexus brachialis, Pars infraclavicularis)

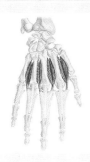

O: sides of the Ossa metacarpi I–V facing each other

I: proximal phalanx and dorsal aponeurosis of the second to fourth fingers

F: metacarpophalangeal joints (II–IV):
• flexion (most important flexors!)
• abduction
interphalangeal joints (II–IV):
• extension

40 Hypothenar muscles

The hypothenar eminence is composed of the M. abductor digiti minimi, M. flexor digiti minimi brevis and the M. opponens digiti minimi (from ulnar to radial). The cutaneous M. palmaris brevis is part of this hypothenar group.

M. palmaris brevis
R. superficialis of the N. ulnaris (Plexus brachialis, Pars infraclavicularis)

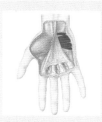

O: Aponeurosis palmaris

I: skin of the hypothenar eminence

F: tenses the skin in the area of the hypothenar eminence

M. abductor digiti minimi
R. profundus of the N. ulnaris (Plexus brachialis, Pars infraclavicularis)

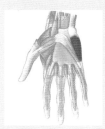

O: Os pisiforme, Retinaculum musculorum flexorum

I: metacarpophalangeal joint V

F: carpometacarpal joint (V):
• opposition
metacarpophalangeal joint (V):
• abduction

M. flexor digiti minimi brevis
R. profundus of the N. ulnaris (Plexus brachialis, Pars infraclavicularis)

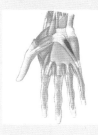

O: Retinaculum musculorum flexorum, Hamulus ossis hamati

I: proximal phalanx of the fifth finger

F: carpometacarpal joint (V):
• opposition
metacarpophalangeal joint (V):
• flexion

M. opponens digiti minimi
R. profundus of the N. ulnaris (Plexus brachialis, Pars infraclavicularis)

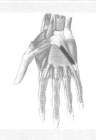

O: Retinaculum musculorum flexorum, Hamulus ossis hamati

I: Os metacarpi V

F: carpometacarpal joint (V):
• opposition

Lower limb

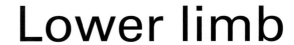

Plexus lumbosacralis
M. iliacus
M. psoas major
M. psoas minor
M. gluteus maximus
M. gluteus medius
M. gluteus minimus
M. tensor fasciae latae
M. piriformis
M. obturatorius internus
M. gemellus superior
M. gemellus inferior
M. quadratus femoris
M. obturatorius externus
M. quadriceps femoris
M. sartorius
M. pectineus
M. gracilis
M. adductor brevis
M. adductor longus
M. adductor magnus
M. biceps femoris
M. semitendinosus
M. semimembranosus
M. tibialis anterior

M. extensor hallucis longus
M. extensor digitorum longus
M. fibularis [peroneus] tertius
M. fibularis [peroneus] longus
M. fibularis [peroneus] brevis
M. triceps surae
M. plantaris
M. popliteus
M. tibialis posterior
M. flexor digitorum longus
M. flexor hallucis longus
M. extensor digitorum brevis
M. extensor hallucis brevis
M. abductor hallucis
M. flexor hallucis brevis
M. adductor hallucis
M. flexor digitorum brevis
M. quadratus plantae
Mm. lumbricales pedis I–IV
Mm. interossei plantares pedis I–III
Mm. interossei dorsales pedis I–IV
M. abductor digiti minimi
M. flexor digiti minimi brevis
M. opponens digiti minimi

Lower limb

41 Joints of the lower limb, Articulationes membri inferioris

41.1 Bony connections of the pelvic girdle, Juncturae cinguli pelvici

Name	Type of connection	Types of movements
Sacroiliac joint Articulatio sacroiliaca	rigid joint, amphiarthrosis	
Ligg. sacroiliaca anteriora Ligg. sacroiliaca posteriora Ligg. sacroiliaca interossea Lig. sacrotuberale Lig. sacrospinale		flexibility and rotation by a few millimeters as a consequence of pelvic deformations caused by various forces
Pubic symphysis, Symphysis pubica	cartilaginous, synchondrosis with Discus interpubicus	
Lig. pubicum superius Lig. pubicum inferius		

41.2 Joints of the free lower limb, Articulationes membri inferioris liberi

Name of joint	Type of joint	Types of movements
Hip joint Articulatio coxae	spheroidal/ball and socket joint, Articulatio spheroidea	• flexion (anteversion) • extension (retroversion) • adduction • abduction • medial rotation • lateral rotation
Knee joint Articulatio genus	pivot (rotary) and ginglymus (hinge) joint, 'trochoginglymus'	• flexion • extension • medial rotation (only possible in a flexed position) • lateral rotation (only possible in a flexed position)
Upper tibiofibular joint Articulatio tibiofibularis	rigid joint, amphiarthrosis	limited sliding movements in transverse and vertical directions as well as limited rotations
Lower tibiofibular connection Syndesmosis tibiofibularis	syndesmosis	embracing of the malleolar mortise; with dorsiflexion in the ankle joint, the malleolar mortise widens slightly
Talocrural (ankle) joint Articulatio talocruralis	hinge joint, ginglymus	• plantar flexion (lowering of the dorsum of the foot) • dorsal extension (elevation of the dorsum of the foot)
Subtalar joint Articulatio talotarsalis a) Articulatio talocalcaneonavicularis (= anterior section) b) Articulatio subtalaris (= posterior section; subtalar)	combined pivot-spheroidal joint spheroidal joint pivot joint	• medial rotation of the hindfoot (= inversion) • lateral rotation of the hindfoot (= eversion) along with CHOPART's and LISFRANC's joints • elevation of the medial margin of the foot (= supination) • elevation of the lateral margin of the foot (= pronation)
Transverse tarsal (midtarsal) joint Articulatio tarsi transversa (CHOPART's joint) a) Articulatio talocalcaneonavicularis b) Articulatio calcaneocuboidea	rigid joint, amphiarthrosis	• torsion of the forefoot • limited plantar and dorsal movements • securing the longitudinal plantar arch of the foot (key joint of the flat foot)
Intertarsal joints a) Articulatio cuneonavicularis b) Articulationes intercuneiformes c) Articulatio cuneocuboidea	rigid joints, amphiarthroses	very restricted movements during adaptive changes of the foot while touching the ground, e.g. when walking
Tarsometatarsal joints Articulationes tarsometatarsales (LISFRANC's joint)	rigid joints, amphiarthroses	• torsion of the forefoot • very limited plantar and dorsal movements

41.2 Joints of the free lower limb, Articulationes membri inferioris liberi (continued)

Name of joint	Type of joint	Types of movements
Intermetatarsal joints Articulationes intermetatarsales	rigid joints, amphiarthroses	very limited movements with torsion of the forefoot
Metatarsophalangeal joints Articulationes metatarsophalangeae	functionally restricted spheroidal joints	• flexion • extension • abduction (straddling toes) • adduction (squeezing toes together)
Interphalangeal joints Articulationes interphalangeae pedis	hinge joints, ginglymi	• flexion • extension of toes

41.3 Planes and axes of movement of joints of the lower limb

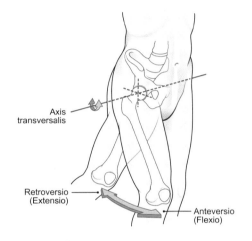

Axis transversalis

Retroversio (Extensio)

Anteversio (Flexio)

Fig. 8 Hip joint;
movement in the sagittal plane. [S700-L126]

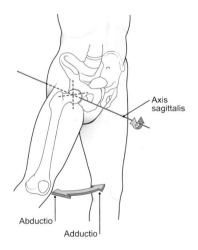

Axis sagittalis

Abductio

Adductio

Fig. 9 Hip joint;
movement in the frontal plane. [S700-L126]

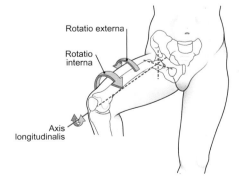

Rotatio externa

Rotatio interna

Axis longitudinalis

Fig. 10 Hip joint;
movement in the transverse plane. [S700-L126]

41.3 Planes and axes of movement of joints of the lower limb (continued)

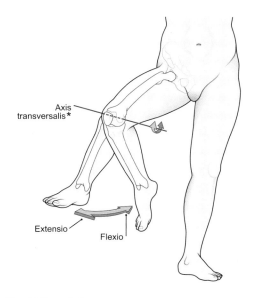

Fig. 11 Knee joint;
movement in the sagittal plane. [S700-L126]
* Due to the uneven curvature of the femoral con-
dyles, the position of this axis changes significantly during movement (instantaneous axis).

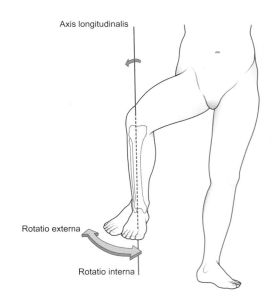

Fig. 12 Knee joint;
movement in the transverse plane. [S700-L126]

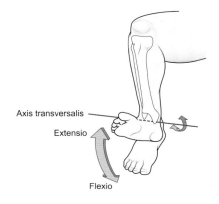

Fig. 13 Talocrural joint;
movement in the sagittal plane. Flexion and extension
movements mainly occur in the talocrural joint. [S700-
L126]

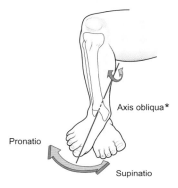

Fig. 14 Subtalar joint;
pronation and supination movements of the foot. [S700-L126]
At maximal plantar flexion, pronation in the Articulatio talocalcaneonavicularis is also referred
to as lateral abduction, and supination as medial abduction.

* The axis projects in a posterior-inferior direction from the medial aspect of the neck of the
talus to the Proc. lateralis of the Tuber calcanei, and is normally steeper than shown here
for didactic reasons.

The plantar flexion in the talocrural joint is also referred to as flexion and the dorsiflexion as extension.

Lower limb

42 Branches and innervation areas of the Plexus lumbosacralis

The **lumbosacral plexus (Plexus lumbosacralis)** is composed of both the Plexus lumbalis and the Plexus sacralis, with their combined nerve fibres forming a lumbosacral network from which individual nerves emerge. In this way, the Truncus lumbosacralis guides the nerve fibres from the L4–5 of the Plexus lumbalis to cross over into the Plexus sacralis. The Rr. anteriores of the spinal nerves from the spinal cord segments T12–L4 form the **Plexus lumbalis** and those from L4–S5 and Co1 form the **Plexus sacralis**. It is important to note that not all spinal cord segments which send fibres into individual nerves of the lumbosacral plexus take part equally in the innervation of all muscles. As certain segments predominate in some muscles, as shown in → Table 43, these can be used as key muscles in clinical diagnostics.

42.1 Branches and supply areas of the Plexus lumbalis

Branch	Motor	Sensory
Rr. musculares T12–L4	Mm. iliopsoas, quadratus lumborum	
N. iliohypogastricus [N. iliopubicus] T12, L1 • R. cutaneus lateralis • R. cutaneus anterior	Mm. rectus abdominis, obliquus internus abdominis, transversus abdominis, pyramidalis, cremaster	• skin above the hip • skin above the iliac crest, the inguinal ligament, and the Mons pubis
N. ilioinguinalis T12, L1 • Nn. scrotales anteriores/ • Nn. labiales anteriores	Mm. rectus abdominis, obliquus internus abdominis, transversus abdominis, pyramidalis, cremaster	• skin in the inguinal region, the root of the penis, the scrotum or the Labia majora
N. genitofemoralis L1, L2 • R. genitalis • R. femoralis		• scrotal layers (including the Tunica dartos) • skin above the Hiatus saphenus
N. cutaneus femoris lateralis L2, L3		• skin on the lateral and anterior side of the thigh down to the knee

N. obturatorius
L2–L4
• R. anterior
  – R. cutaneus
• R. posterior
  – Rr. musculares
	Mm. obturatorius externus, pectineus, adductor longus, adductor brevis, adductor magnus, gracilis	• capsule of the hip joint
		• skin at the medial aspect of the thigh above the knee
		• capsule of the hip joint, periosteum at the posterior side of the thigh

N. femoralis
L2–L4
• Rr. musculares
• Rr. cutanei anteriores
• N. saphenus
  – R. infrapatellaris
  – Rr. cutanei cruris mediales
	Mm. iliopsoas, pectineus, sartorius, quadriceps femoris	• capsule of the hip joint
		• skin of the anterior and medial sides of the thigh down to the knee, periosteum of the anterior side of the thigh
		• skin of the medial and anterior sides of the knee and on the medial side of the leg and the foot

42.2 Branches and innervation areas of the Plexus sacralis

Branch	Motor	Sensory
N. musculi obturatorii interni L5–S2	Mm. obturatorius internus, gemellus superior	
N. musculi piriformis S1, S2	M. piriformis	
N. musculi quadrati femoris L4–S1	Mm. quadratus femoris, gemellus inferior	
N. gluteus superior L4–S1	Mm. glutei medius and minimus, tensor fasciae latae	
N. gluteus inferior L5–S2	M. gluteus maximus	

Lower limb

42.2 Branches and innervation areas of the Plexus sacralis (continued)

Branch	Motor	Sensory
N. cutaneus femoris posterior S1–S3 • Nn. clunium inferiores • Nn. perineales		• skin on the posterior side of the thigh and the proximal lower limb • skin of the gluteal region • perineum, scrotal skin or skin of the Labia majora
N. ischiadicus L4–S3	ischiocrural (hamstring) muscles, all muscles of the lower limb and foot	
N. fibularis communis L4–S2 • N. cutaneus surae lateralis • R. communicans fibularis	M. biceps femoris, Caput breve	• capsule of the knee joint • skin of the calf up to the lateral malleolus • connecting branch to the N. suralis
N. fibularis superficialis L4–S2 • Rr. musculares • N. cutaneus dorsalis medialis • N. cutaneus dorsalis intermedius • Nn. digitales dorsales pedis	Mm. fibulares [peronei] longus and brevis	• skin of the lower limb and dorsum of the foot up to the first to third toes • skin of the lower limb and dorsum of the foot between the third and fifth toes (medial side) • skin of the dorsum of the toes with the exception of the first interdigital space and the lateral side of the fifth toe
N. fibularis profundus L4–S2 • Rr. musculares • Nn. digitales dorsales pedis	Mm. tibialis anterior, extensor digitorum longus, extensor hallucis longus, extensor digitorum brevis and extensor hallucis brevis	periosteum of the leg bones and capsule of the talocrural joint skin of the first interdigital space

N. tibialis
L4–S3
• Rr. musculares
• N. interosseus cruris
• N. cutaneus surae medialis
• N. suralis
  – N. cutaneus dorsalis lateralis
  – Rr. calcanei laterales
  – Rr. calcanei mediales
• N. plantaris medialis
  – Nn. digitales plantares communes
    – Nn. digitales plantares proprii
• N. plantaris lateralis
  – R. superficialis
    – Nn. digitales plantares communes
    – Nn. digitales plantares proprii
  – R. profundus
	Mm. triceps surae, plantaris, popliteus, tibialis posterior, flexor digitorum longus, flexor hallucis longus
	Mm. abductor hallucis and flexor digitorum brevis, flexor hallucis brevis (medial head), lumbricales pedis I (II)
	Mm. abductor digiti minimi, quadratus plantae
	Mm. flexor digiti minimi brevis, opponens digiti minimi, interossei
	Mm. lumbricales pedis II–IV, adductor hallucis (Caput transversum)
		• capsule of the knee joint
		• periosteum of the lower limb bones and capsule of the talocrural joint
		• skin of the calf up to the medial malleolus
		• joins the N. cutaneus surae lateralis to form the N. suralis
		• skin of the lateral margin of the foot up to the lateral aspect of the fifth toe
		• skin of the heel, lateral aspect
		• skin of the heel, medial aspect
		• skin of the medial margin of the foot
		• skin of the plantar side of the medial 3½ toes and their nail areas
		• skin on the plantar side of the lateral 1½ toes and their nail areas

N. cutaneus perforans S2–S3		pierces the Lig. sacrotuberale and innervates the overlying skin area

N. pudendus
S2–S4
• Nn. rectales [anales] inferiores
  S3, S4
• Nn. perineales
  – Nn. scrotales posteriores
  – Nn. labiales posteriores
  – Rr. musculares
  – N. dorsalis penis/N. dorsalis clitoridis
	Mm. transversi perinei superficialis and profundus, bulbospongiosus and ischiocavernosus, sphincter ani externus	• skin of the anal region and the perineum
		• mucosa of the urethra, dorsal scrotal skin or posterior areas of the Labia majora and minora, Vestibulum vaginae
		• skin of the penis, glans/clitoris, prepuce

Rr. musculares S3, S4	Mm. levator ani, ischiococcygeus	
N. anococcygeus S5–Co1		skin above the coccyx and the region between the coccyx and anus

43 Segmental innervation of muscles of the lower limb, diagnostically significant key muscles

The muscles printed in bold are used clinically as key muscles for specific segments.

Segmental innervation of muscles of the lower limb, diagnostically significant key muscles

M. iliopsoas: L1, L2	T12–L3	**M. tibialis anterior: L4**	L4–L5
M. tensor fasciae latae	L4–L5	**M. extensor hallucis longus: L5**	L4–S1
M. gluteus medius	L4–S1	M. popliteus	L4–S1
M. gluteus minimus	L4–S1	**M. extensor digitorum longus: L5**	L4–S1
M. gluteus maximus	L4–S2	**M. soleus**	L4–S2
M. obturatorius internus	L5–S1	**M. gastrocnemius** } S1	
M. piriformis	L5–S1	M. fibularis [peroneus] longus	L5–S1
M. sartorius	L2–L3	M. fibularis [peroneus] brevis	L5–S1
M. pectineus	L2–L3	**M. tibialis posterior: S1**	L5–S2
M. adductor longus	L2–L3	M. flexor digitorum longus	L5–S3
M. quadriceps femoris: L3	L2–L4	M. flexor hallucis longus	L5–S3
M. gracilis	L2–L4	M. extensor hallucis brevis	L4–S1
M. adductor brevis	L2–L4	M. extensor digitorum brevis	L4–S1
M. obturatorius externus	L3–L4	M. flexor digitorum brevis	L5–S1
M. adductor magnus	L3–L4	M. abductor hallucis	L5–S1
M. semitendinosus	L4–S1	M. flexor hallucis brevis	L5–S3
M. semimembranosus	L4–S1	M. adductor hallucis	S1–S2
M. biceps femoris	L4–S2		

44 Ventral muscles of the hip

The M. iliopsoas, which is composed of the M. iliacus and M. psoas major, is the only muscle in this group, because it is the only ventral muscle of the lower limb which exclusively crosses the hip joint. All other muscles located in front of the hip joint also span the knee joint and are therefore collectively referred to as muscles of the thigh.

M. iliacus (part of M. iliopsoas)
Rr. musculares (Plexus lumbalis)

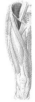

I: Fossa iliaca

I: Trochanter minor

F: lumbar vertebral column:
- lateroflexion
hip joint:
- flexion (most important muscle)
- lateral rotation from a medial rotational position

M. psoas major (part of the M. iliopsoas)
Rr. musculares (Plexus lumbalis)

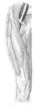

O: superficial layer: lateral surface of the bodies of the thoracic to lumbar vertebrae T12 to L4, Disci intervertebrales
deep layer: Proc. costalis of the lumbar vertebrae L1–L4

I: Trochanter minor and adjacent area of the Labium mediale of the Linea aspera

F: lumbar vertebral column:
- lateroflexion
hip joint:
- flexion (most important muscle)
- lateral rotation from a medial rotational position

M. psoas minor (part of M. iliopsoas; inconstant; often ends in a long flat tendon)
Rr. musculares (Plexus lumbalis)

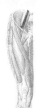

O: lateral surface of the bodies of the thoracic and lumbar vertebrae T12 and L1

I: fascia of the M. iliopsoas, Arcus iliopectineus

F: lumbar vertebral column:
- lateroflexion

Lower limb

45 Dorsolateral muscles of the hip

The M. gluteus maximus shapes the surface of the gluteal region significantly and covers the other muscles of this group almost completely. Ventrocranially the M. gluteus medius is visible, which in turn covers the M. gluteus minimus. The M. piriformis, M. gemellus superior, M. obturatorius internus, M. gemellus inferior, M. quadratus femoris and M. obturatorius externus follow caudally and deep inside.
The M. obturatorius internus, M. gemellus superior and M. gemellus inferior are collectively named the M. triceps coxae. The most laterally located M. tensor fasciae latae with its short muscle belly projects into the Tractus iliotibialis.

M. gluteus maximus
N. gluteus inferior (Plexus sacralis)

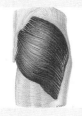

O: Facies glutea of the Os ilium dorsal to the Linea glutea posterior, Facies posterior of the Os sacrum, Fascia thoracolumbalis, Lig. sacrotuberale

I: cranial part: Tractus iliotibialis caudal part: Tuberositas glutea

F: hip joint:
- extension (most important muscle)
- lateral rotation (most important muscle)
- cranial part: abduction
- caudal part: adduction

knee joint:
- stabilisation in the extended position
- tension band effect on the femur

M. gluteus medius
N. gluteus superior (Plexus sacralis)

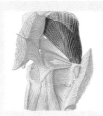

O: Facies glutea of the Os ilium between the Lineae gluteae anterior and posterior

I: tip of the Trochanter major

F: hip joint:
- abduction (most important muscle)

ventral part:
- flexion
- medial rotation (most important muscle)

dorsal part:
- extension
- lateral rotation

M. gluteus minimus
N. gluteus superior (Plexus sacralis)

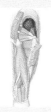

O: Facies glutea of the Os ilium between the Lineae gluteae anterior and inferior

I: tip of the Trochanter major

F: hip joint:
- abduction

ventral part:
- flexion
- medial rotation

dorsal part:
- extension
- lateral rotation

M. tensor fasciae latae
N. gluteus superior (Plexus lumbosacralis)

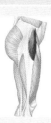

O: Spina iliaca anterior superior

I: via the Tractus iliotibialis, at the tibia below the Condylus lateralis

F: hip joint:
- flexion
- abduction
- medial rotation

knee joint:
- stabilisation in the extended position
- tension band effect on the femur

Lower limb

46 Pelvitrochanteric muscles of the hip

M. piriformis
(Rr. musculares) Plexus sacralis

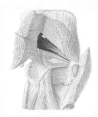

I: Facies pelvica of the Os sacrum

I: tip of the Trochanter major

F: hip joint:
- lateral rotation
- abduction

M. obturatorius internus
(Rr. musculares) Plexus sacralis

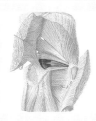

O: bony rim of the Foramen obturatum, medial area of the Membrana obturatoria

I: tip of the Trochanter major

F: hip joint:
- lateral rotation

M. gemellus superior
(Rr. musculares) Plexus sacralis

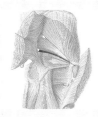

O: Spina ischiadica

I: tendon of the M. obturatorius internus

F: hip joint:
- lateral rotation

M. gemellus inferior
(Rr. musculares) Plexus sacralis

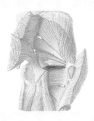

O: Tuber ischiadicum

I: tendon of the M. obturatorius internus

F: hip joint:
- lateral rotation

M. quadratus femoris
(Rr. musculares) Plexus sacralis

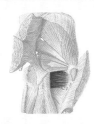

O: Tuber ischiadicum

I: Crista intertrochanterica

F: hip joint:
- lateral rotation
- adduction

→ Table 46 Pelvitrochanteric muscles of the hip

M. obturatorius externus
N. obturatorius (Plexus lumbalis)

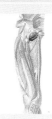

O: bony rim of the Foramen obturatum, lateral area of the Membrana obturatoria

I: Fossa trochanterica

F: hip joint:
- lateral rotation
- adduction

47 Ventral muscles of the thigh

The M. sartorius crosses the thigh in an oblique direction from proximal lateral to distal medial. The M. quadriceps femoris constitutes the largest part of the muscles located ventrally on the thigh.

M. quadriceps femoris
N. femoralis (Plexus lumbalis)

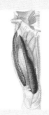

O: M. rectus femoris: Spina iliaca anterior inferior,
cranial rim of the acetabulum
M. vastus medialis: Labium mediale of the Linea aspera
M. vastus lateralis: Trochanter major, Labium laterale of the Linea aspera
M. vastus intermedius: Facies anterior of the femur

I: Patella,
Tuberositas tibiae via Lig. patellae, areas to both sides of the Tuberositas tibiae via Retinacula patellae

F: hip joint: (only M. rectus femoris):
- flexion
knee joint:
- extension (unique extensor!)

M. sartorius
N. femoralis (Plexus lumbalis)

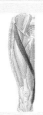

O: Spina iliaca anterior superior

I: Condylus medialis of the tibia (superficial Pes anserinus)

F: hip joint:
- flexion
- lateral rotation
- abduction
knee joint:
- flexion
- medial rotation

48 Medial muscles of the thigh (adductors)

The M. gracilis is positioned furthest medially. The M. pectineus, M. adductor brevis, M. adductor longus and M. adductor magnus are arranged from proximal to distal.

M. pectineus
N. femoralis and N. obturatorius (Plexus lumbalis)

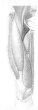

O: Pecten ossis pubis

I: Trochanter minor and Linea pectinea of the femur

F: hip joint:
- adduction
- flexion
- lateral rotation

M. gracilis
N. obturatorius (Plexus lumbalis)

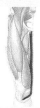

O: Corpus ossis pubis, Ramus inferior ossis pubis

I: Condylus medialis of the tibia (superficial Pes anserinus)

F: hip joint:
- adduction
- flexion
- lateral rotation

knee joint:
- flexion
- medial rotation

M. adductor brevis
N. obturatorius (Plexus lumbalis)

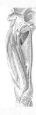

O: Ramus inferior ossis pubis

I: proximal third of the Labium mediale of the Linea aspera

F: hip joint:
- adduction
- flexion
- lateral rotation

M. adductor longus
N. obturatorius (Plexus lumbalis)

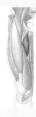

O: Os pubis up to the Symphysis pubica

I: middle third of the Labium mediale of the Linea aspera

F: hip joint:
- adduction
- flexion
- lateral rotation

M. adductor magnus (An incomplete proximal separation of the M. adductor magnus is called the M. adductor minimus.)
Main part: N. obturatorius (Plexus lumbalis); dorsal part: tibial division of the N. ischiadicus (Plexus sacralis)

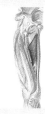

O: main part:
Ramus inferior ossis pubis, Ramus ossis ischii
dorsal part:
Tuber ischiadicum

I: proximal two-thirds of the Labium mediale of the Linea aspera, Epicondylus medialis of the femur, Septum intermusculare vastoadductorium

F: hip joint:
- adduction
- lateral rotation

main part:
- flexion

dorsal part:
- extension

Lower limb

49 Dorsal muscles of the thigh (ischiocrural muscles)

The M. biceps femoris, M. semitendinosus, and M. semimembranosus (from lateral to medial) constitute the dorsal muscles of the thigh.

M. biceps femoris (Caput longum: crossing two joints, Caput breve: crossing one joint)
Caput longum: N. ischiadicus, tibial division (Plexus sacralis)
Caput breve: N. ischiadicus, fibular division (Plexus sacralis)

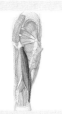

O: Caput longum: Tuber ischiadicum
Caput breve: middle third of the Labium laterale of the Linea aspera

I: Caput fibulae

F: hip joint:
- extension
- lateral rotation
- adduction

knee joint:
- flexion
- lateral rotation (most important muscle)

M. semitendinosus
Tibial part of the N. ischiadicus (Plexus sacralis)

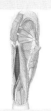

O: Tuber ischiadicum

I: Condylus medialis of the tibia (superficial Pes anserinus)

F: hip joint:
- extension
- medial rotation

knee joint:
- flexion
- medial rotation

M. semimembranosus
Tibial part of the N. ischiadicus (Plexus sacralis)

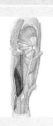

O: Tuber ischiadicum

I: Condylus medialis of the tibia (deep Pes anserinus)

F: hip joint:
- extension
- medial rotation

knee joint:
- flexion (most important muscle)
- medial rotation (most important muscle)

50 Ventral muscles of the lower limb

The M. tibialis anterior runs the most superficially and medially of all the muscles. The M. extensor digitorum longus follows laterally, frequently generating the M. fibularis tertius at its lateral margin. The M. extensor hallucis longus is located furthest distally.

M. tibialis anterior
N. fibularis profundus (N. ischiadicus)

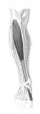

O: Facies lateralis of the tibia, Fascia cruris, Membrana interossea

I: Os metatarsi I, Os cuneiforme mediale

F: talocrural joint:
- dorsiflexion (most important muscle)

subtalar joint:
- supination (weak)

M. extensor hallucis longus
N. fibularis profundus (N. ischiadicus)

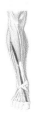

O: Facies medialis of the fibula, Membrana interossea, Fascia cruris

I: Phalanx distalis of the hallux

F: talocrural joint:
- dorsiflexion

subtalar joint:
- pronation (weak)

joints of the hallux:
- extension

M. extensor digitorum longus
N. fibularis profundus (N. ischiadicus)

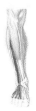

O: Condylus lateralis of the tibia, Margo anterior of the fibula, Membrana interossea cruris, Fascia cruris

I: dorsal aponeuroses of the second to the fifth toes

F: talocrural joint:
- dorsiflexion

subtalar joint:
- pronation

interphalangeal joints:
- extension

M. fibularis [peroneus] tertius (inconstant muscle)
N. fibularis profundus (N. ischiadicus)

O: distal separation of the M. extensor digitorum longus

I: Os metatarsi V

F: talocrural joint:
- dorsiflexion

subtalar joint:
- pronation

Lower limb

51 Lateral (fibular) muscles of the lower limb

The M. fibularis longus is located superficially and laterally, and distally thereof lies the M. fibularis brevis.

M. fibularis [peroneus] longus
N. fibularis superficialis (N. ischiadicus)

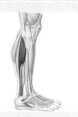

O: Caput fibulae, proximal two-thirds of the fibula, Fascia cruris | **I:** Tuberositas ossis metatarsi I, Os cuneiforme mediale | **F: talocrural joint:**
- plantar flexion

subtalar joint:
- pronation (most important muscle)

M. fibularis [peroneus] brevis
N. fibularis superficialis (N. ischiadicus)

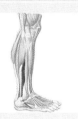

O: distal half of the fibula | **I:** Tuberositas ossis metatarsi V | **F: talocrural joint:**
- plantar flexion

subtalar joint:
- pronation

52 Dorsal superficial muscles of the lower limb

The surface of the calf is shaped by the heads of the M. gastrocnemius. This muscle is located superficially to the M. soleus and together they constitute the M. triceps surae. The very small M. plantaris can be considered as the fourth head of this muscle.

M. triceps surae (The broad tendon of the M. triceps surae is known as the ACHILLES tendon.)
N. tibialis (N. ischiadicus)

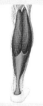

O: M. gastrocnemius, Caput mediale: Condylus medialis of the femur
M. gastrocnemius, Caput laterale: Condylus lateralis of the femur
M. soleus: proximal third of the fibula, Facies posterior of the tibia (Linea musculi solei), Arcus tendineus musculi solei | **I:** Tuber calcanei | **F: knee joint** (only M. gastrocnemius and M. plantaris):
- flexion

talocrural joint:
- plantar flexion (most important muscle)

subtalar joint:
- supination (most important muscle)

M. plantaris
N. tibialis (N. ischiadicus)

O: Condylus lateralis of the femur | **I:** Tuber calcanei | **F: knee joint:**
- flexion

talocrural joint:
- plantar flexion

subtalar joint:
- supination

53 Dorsal deep muscles of the lower limb

The M. popliteus is the most proximal muscle and runs in a lateral oblique direction to the knee joint. The M. tibialis posterior lies in the middle of the muscles running to the foot, accompanied by the M. flexor digitorum longus on its medial side and the M. flexor hallucis longus on its lateral side.

M. popliteus
N. tibialis (N. ischiadicus)

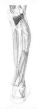

O: Condylus lateralis of the femur, posterior horn of the lateral meniscus

I: Facies posterior of the tibia, superior to the Linea musculi solei

F: knee joint:
* medial rotation
* prevents entrapment of the meniscus

M. tibialis posterior
N. tibialis (N. ischiadicus)

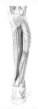

O: Membrana interossea, tibia and fibula

I: Tuberositas ossis navicularis, plantar surface of the Ossa cuneiformia I–III, Ossa metatarsi II–IV

F: talocrural joint:
* plantar flexion

subtalar joint:
* supination (second most important muscle)

M. flexor digitorum longus
N. tibialis (N. ischiadicus)

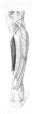

O: Facies posterior of the tibia

I: Phalanx distalis of the second to fifth toes

F: talocrural joint:
* plantar flexion

subtalar joint:
* supination

interphalangeal joints of the toes:
* flexion

M. flexor hallucis longus
N. tibialis (N. ischiadicus)

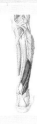

O: distal Facies posterior to the fibula, Membrana interossea

I: Phalanx distalis of the hallux

F: talocrural joint:
* plantar flexion

subtalar joint:
* supination

joints of the hallux:
* flexion

54 Muscles of the dorsum of the foot

The two muscles are only faintly visible under the skin of the dorsum of the foot. The M. extensor hallucis brevis runs to the hallux (big toe), and the M. extensor digitorum brevis runs to the other toes.

M. extensor digitorum brevis
N. fibularis profundus (N. ischiadicus)

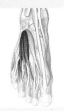

| **O:** dorsal aspect of the calcaneus | **I:** dorsal aponeurosis of the second to fourth toes | **F: interphalangeal joints of the toes** (II–IV):
 • extension |

M. extensor hallucis brevis
N. fibularis profundus (N. ischiadicus)

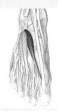

| **O:** dorsal aspect of the calcaneus | **I:** Phalanx proximalis of the hallux | **F: metatarsophalangeal joint of the hallux:**
 • extension |

55 Medial muscles of the sole of the foot

The M. abductor hallucis is mainly responsible for the surface of the medial margin of the foot. Adjacent lies the M. flexor hallucis brevis, and laterally follows the M. adductor hallucis.

M. abductor hallucis
N. plantaris medialis (N. tibialis)

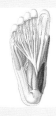

| **O:** Proc. medialis of the Tuber calcanei, Aponeurosis plantaris, Retinaculum musculorum flexorum | **I:** medial sesamoid bone of the metatarsophalangeal joint, Phalanx proximalis of the hallux | **F: metatarsophalangeal joint of the hallux:**
 • abduction
 • flexion <br> bracing of the medial longitudinal plantar arch |

M. flexor hallucis brevis
Caput mediale: N. plantaris medialis (N. tibialis)
Caput laterale: N. plantaris lateralis (N. tibialis)

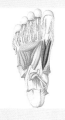

| **O:** plantar aspect of the Ossa cuneiformia, plantar ligaments | **I: Caput mediale:** medial sesamoid bone of the metatarsophalangeal joint, Phalanx proximalis of the hallux
 Caput laterale: lateral sesamoid bone of the metatarsophalangeal joint, Phalanx proximalis of the hallux | **F: metatarsophalangeal joint of the hallux:**
 • flexion <br> bracing of the longitudinal plantar arch |

M. adductor hallucis
N. plantaris lateralis (N. tibialis)

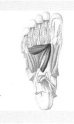

| **O: Caput obliquum:** Os cuboideum, Os cuneiforme, plantar ligaments
 Caput transversum: capsules of the metatarsophalangeal joints of the third to fifth toes, Lig. metatarsale transversum profundum | **I:** lateral sesamoid bone and capsule of the metatarsophalangeal joint I, Phalanx proximalis of the hallux | **F: metatarsophalangeal joint of the hallux:**
 • adduction towards the second toe
 • flexion <br> bracing of the longitudinal and transverse plantar arches |

56 Muscles in the middle of the sole of the foot

In its proximal part, the M. flexor digitorum brevis is firmly attached to the plantar aponeurosis. Beneath this muscle, the M. quadratus plantae connects with the main tendon of the M. flexor digitorum longus. The Mm. lumbricales pedis I–IV originate from its four tendinous branches. The Mm. interossei plantares I–III and the Mm. interossei dorsales pedis I–IV fill the spaces between the Ossa metatarsi.

M. flexor digitorum brevis (Shortly before their insertion point, the tendons of this muscle are pierced by the tendons of the M. flexor digitorum longus.)
N. plantaris medialis (N. tibialis)

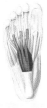

O: plantar aspect of the Tuber calcanei, Aponeurosis plantaris

I: middle phalanx of the second to the fifth toes

F: metatarsophalangeal and proximal interphalangeal joints of the toes:
- flexion
bracing of the longitudinal plantar arch

M. quadratus plantae
N. plantaris lateralis (N. tibialis)

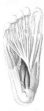

O: plantar aspect of the calcaneus, Lig. plantare longum

I: lateral margin of the tendon of the M. flexor digitorum longus

F: supports the M. flexor digitorum longus

Mm. lumbricales pedis I–IV
Nn. plantares medialis (I) and lateralis (II–IV) (N. tibialis)

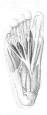

O: M. lumbricalis pedis: tendons of the M. flexor digitorum longus
I: single-headed
II–IV: two-headed

I: medial side of the Phalanx proximalis of the second to fifth toes

F: metatarsophalangeal joints of the toes:
- flexion
- adduction

Mm. interossei plantares pedis I–III
N. plantaris lateralis (N. tibialis)

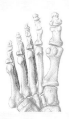

O: plantar aspect of the Ossa metatarsi III–V, Lig. plantare longum

I: medial side of the Phalanx proximalis of the third to fifth toes

F: metatarsophalangeal joints of the toes:
- flexion
- adduction towards the second toe

Mm. interossei dorsales pedis I–IV (two-headed muscles)
N. plantaris lateralis (N. tibialis)

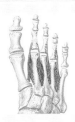

O: sides of the Ossa metatarsi I–V facing each other, Lig. plantare longum

I: Phalanx proximalis of the second to fourth toes (second toe bilateral, third and fourth toes from lateral)

F: metatarsophalangeal joints of the toes:
- flexion
- medial abduction of the second toe, lateral abduction of the third and fourth toes

Lower limb

57 Lateral muscles of the sole of the foot

The M. abductor digiti minimi runs along the lateral margin of the foot. Beneath its plantar surface lie the M. flexor digiti minimi brevis and the M. opponens digiti minimi.

M. abductor digiti minimi
N. plantaris lateralis (N. tibialis)

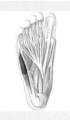

O: Proc. lateralis of the Tuber calcanei, Aponeurosis plantaris

I: Tuberositas ossis metatarsi V, Phalanx proximalis of the fifth toe

F: metatarsophalangeal joints of the toes:
- abduction
- flexion

bracing of the longitudinal plantar arch

M. flexor digiti minimi brevis
N. plantaris lateralis (N. tibialis)

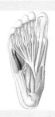

O: base of the Os metatarsi V, Lig. plantare longum

I: Phalanx proximalis of the fifth toe

F: metatarsophalangeal joints of the toes:
- flexion

bracing of the longitudinal plantar arch

M. opponens digiti minimi (inconstant muscle)
N. plantaris lateralis (N. tibialis)

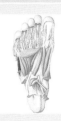

O: base of the Os metatarsi V, Lig. plantare longum

I: Os metatarsi V

F: metatarsophalangeal joints of the toes:
- opposition

bracing of the longitudinal plantar arch

Cranial nerves

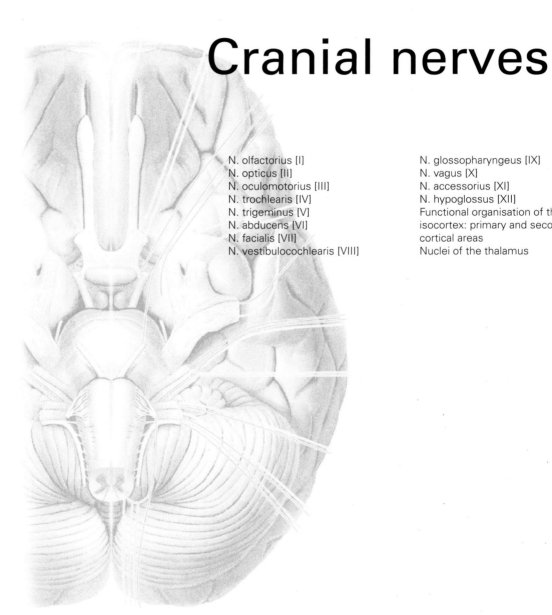

58 Cranial nerves, overview

a	**N. olfactorius [I]**
b	**N. opticus [II]**
c	**N. oculomotorius [III]**
d	**N. trochlearis [IV]**
e	**N. trigeminus [V]** • N. ophthalmicus [V/1] • N. maxillaris [V/2] • N. mandibularis [V/3]
f	**N. abducens [VI]**
g	**N. facialis [VII]**
h	**N. vestibulocochlearis [VIII]**
i	**N. glossopharyngeus [IX]**
j	**N. vagus [X]**
k	**N. accessorius [XI]**
l	**N. hypoglossus [XII]**

59 Cranial nerves, functions (fibre qualities)

(GSE)	General somatic-efferent: innervation of the skeletal muscles **(III, IV, VI, XII)**
(GVE)	General visceral-efferent: innervation of visceral and vascular smooth muscles and glands **(III, VII, IX, X)**
(SVE)	Special visceral-efferent: innervation of the facial muscles, masticatory muscles, larynx, pharynx, oesophagus, M. sternocleidomastoideus, M. trapezius **(V, VII, IX, X, XI)**
(GVA)	General visceral-afferent: information from viscera and blood vessels **(IX, X)**
(SVA)	Special visceral-afferent: taste **(VII, IX, X)**
(GSA)	General somatic-afferent: pain, temperature, information via mechanoreceptors of the skin and musculoskeletal system **(V, VII, IX, X)**
(SSA)	Special somatic-afferent: smell, vision, hearing, equilibrium/balance **(VIII)**

60 Cranial nerves

60.1 N. olfactorius [I]

The Fila olfactoria are collectively known as the N. olfactorius. They constitute the peripheral neuron of the olfactory pathway.

Origin	olfactory cells of the Regio olfactoria
Passage through the cranial base	Lamina cribrosa
Passage through the dura mater	Lamina cribrosa
Entry point into the brain	Bulbus olfactorius
Innervation areas	mucosa (olfactory epithelium) at the roof of the nasal cavity, the upper nasal concha and the upper part of the nasal septum

60.2 N. opticus [II]

The N. opticus is not a peripheral nerve but a part of the diencephalon.

Origin	Stratum ganglionare of the retina
Pathway in the dura mater	Vagina nervi optici
Passage through the cranial base	Canalis opticus
Other visible pathway	Chiasma opticum, continuation of fibres in the Tractus opticus, Corpus geniculatum laterale
Innervation area	retina

60.3 N. oculomotorius [III]

Nuclei (quality)	• Nucleus nervi oculomotorii (paired main and unpaired accessory nucleus) (GSE) • Nucleus accessorius nervi oculomotorii (GVE) → Ganglion ciliare
Exit point from the brain	Fossa interpeduncularis of the mesencephalon
Location in the subarachnoid space	Cisterna basalis, Cisterna interpeduncularis
Entry point into the dura mater	roof of the Sinus cavernosus
Exit point from the dura mater	Fissura orbitalis superior
Passage through the cranial base	Fissura orbitalis superior (medial part, within the Anulus tendineus)
Innervation areas	**motor:** M. levator palpebrae superioris, Mm. recti superior, medialis and inferior, M. obliquus inferior **parasympathetic:** M. ciliaris, M. sphincter pupillae (via Ganglion ciliare)
Adjunct nerves	**sensory fibres** of the N. nasociliaris (V/1) **sympathetic fibres** of the Plexus ophthalmicus

60.4 N. trochlearis [IV]

Nucleus (quality)	Nucleus nervi trochlearis (GSE)
Exit point from the brain	dorsal, caudal of the Colliculus inferior (Tectum mesencephali)
Location in the subarachnoid space	Cisterna ambiens, Cisterna basalis
Entry point into the dura mater	gap between the Plicae petroclinoideae anterior and posterior
Pathway within the dura mater	lateral wall of the Sinus cavernosus
Exit point from the dura mater	Fissura orbitalis superior
Passage through the cranial base	Fissura orbitalis superior (lateral part)
Innervation area	**motor:** M. obliquus superior

60.5 N. trigeminus [V]

Nuclei (quality)	• Nucleus mesencephalicus nervi trigemini (GSA) • Nucleus pontinus nervi trigemini (Nucleus principalis nervi trigemini) (GSA) • Nucleus spinalis nervi trigemini (GSA) • Nucleus motorius nervi trigemini (SVE)
Exit point from the brain	lateral margin of the pons
Location in the subarachnoid space	Cisterna basalis, Cavum trigeminale
Entry point into the dura mater	as Ganglion trigeminale in the lateral wall of the Sinus cavernosus
Division into three branches	• N. ophthalmicus [V/1] • N. maxillaris [V/2] • N. mandibularis [V/3]

N. ophthalmicus [V/1]

Pathway within the dura mater	lateral wall of the Sinus cavernosus
Exit point from the dura mater	Fissura orbitalis superior
Exit point from the cranial base	Fissura orbitalis superior • N. nasociliaris: medial part • N. frontalis: lateral part • N. lacrimalis: lateral part
Innervation areas	**sensory:** dura mater of the anterior cranial fossa, Falx cerebri, Tentorium cerebelli, forehead. upper eyelid, dorsum of the nose, sclera, cornea, Cellulae ethmoidales anteriores, Sinus sphenoidalis, nasal cavity (anterior part)

N. maxillaris [V/2]

Pathway within the dura mater	lateral wall of the Sinus cavernosus
Exit point from the dura mater	Foramen rotundum
Exit point from the cranial base	Foramen rotundum
Innervation areas	**sensory:** dura mater of the Fossa cranii media, cheek, lower eyelid, lateral surface of the nose, upper lip, teeth and gingiva of the maxilla, Cellulae ethmoidales posteriores, Sinus sphenoidalis, Sinus maxillaris, Conchae nasales superior and media, Palatum, Tonsilla palatina, pharynx (roof)
Adjunct nerves	**parasympathetic (secretory) fibres** to divergent Rr. nasales for the <u>Glandulae nasales</u>, the Nn. palatini for the <u>Glandulae palatinae</u> as well as to the N. zygomaticus for the <u>Glandula lacrimalis</u> (derived from the Nucleus salivatorius superior via N. facialis, N. petrosus major, and Rr. ganglionares to the Ganglion pterygopalatinum, N. zygomaticus, R. communicans cum nervo zygomatico, N. lacrimalis)

N. mandibularis [V/3]

Pathway within the dura mater	lateral wall of the Sinus cavernosus
Exit point from the dura mater	Foramen ovale
Exit point from the cranial base	Foramen ovale
Innervation areas	**motor:** masticatory muscles, M. tensor veli palatini, M. mylohyoideus, M. digastricus (Venter anterior), M. tensor tympani **sensory:** dura mater of the Fossa cranii media, Cellulae mastoideae, skin of the mandible, temple, cheek, auricle (upper part), external acoustic meatus, Membrana tympanica (outer surface), teeth and gingiva of the mandible, anterior two-thirds of the tongue, Isthmus faucium, temporomandibular joint
Adjunct nerves	**sensory:** anterior two-thirds of the tongue (from N. facialis [VII] via Chorda tympani to N. lingualis) **parasympathetic (secretory) fibres** a) to the N. lingualis for the Glandulae submandibularis and sublingualis (from Nucleus salivatorius superior via N. facialis and Chorda tympani to the Ganglion submandibulare) b) to the N. auriculotemporalis for the Glandula parotidea (from Nucleus salivatorius inferior via N. glosso-pharyngeus, N. tympanicus, Plexus tympanicus, and N. petrosus minor to the Ganglion oticum)

60.6 N. abducens [VI]

Nucleus (quality)	Nucleus nervi abducentis (GSE)
Exit point from the brain	between pons and pyramis
Location in the subarachnoid space	Cisterna basalis
Entry point into the dura mater	upper third of the Clivus
Pathway within the dura mater	freely passing through the Sinus cavernosus, lateral to the A. carotis interna
Exit point from the dura mater	Fissura orbitalis superior
Passage through the cranial base	Fissura orbitalis superior, medial part (within the Anulus tendineus)
Innervation area	**motor:** M. rectus lateralis

60.7 N. facialis [VII]

Nuclei (quality)	• Nucleus nervi facialis (SVE) • Nucleus salivatorius superior (GVE) 　– Ganglion pterygopalatinum 　– Ganglion submandibulare • Nucleus solitarius (SVA) • Nucleus spinalis nervi trigemini (GSA)
Exit point from the brain	cerebellopontine angle
Location in the subarachnoid space	Cisterna basalis, Cisterna pontocerebellaris
Entry point into the cranial base	Porus → Meatus acusticus internus
Passage through the dura mater	Fundus meatus acustici interni
Pathway inside the cranial base	Canalis nervi facialis
Exit point from the cranial base	Foramen stylomastoideum
Innervation areas	**motor:** facial (mimic) muscles, Mm. auriculares, M. digastricus (Venter posterior), M. stylohyoideus, M. stapedius **sensory:** anterior two-thirds of the tongue (via Chorda tympani to the N. lingualis) **parasympathetic:** Glandula lacrimalis, Glandulae nasales, Glandulae palatinae (via Ganglion pterygopalatinum), Glandula submandibularis, Glandula sublingualis (via Ganglion submandibulare)
Adjunct nerves	**sensory fibres** of the N. trigeminus to the facial branches of the N. facialis

60.8 N. vestibulocochlearis [VIII]

Nuclei (quality)	• Nuclei cochleares anterior and posterior (SSA) • Nuclei vestibulares medialis, lateralis, superior and inferior (SSA)
Exit point from the brain	cerebellopontine angle
Location in the subarachnoid space	Cisterna basalis, Cisterna pontocerebellaris
Entry point into the cranial base	Porus → Meatus acusticus internus
Exit point from the dura mater	Fundus meatus acustici interni
Pathway inside the cranial base	directly to the labyrinth within the petrous part of the temporal bone
Innervation areas	**sensory:** N. cochlearis: acoustic organ (= CORTI's organ) **sensory:** N. vestibularis: equilibrium/vestibular organ

60.9 N. glossopharyngeus [IX]

Nuclei (quality)	• Nucleus ambiguus (SVE) • Nucleus solitarius (SVA and GVA) • Nucleus salivatorius inferior (GVE) → Ganglion oticum • Nucleus spinalis nervi trigemini (GSA)
Exit point from the brain	Medulla oblongata: Sulcus retroolivaris
Location in the subarachnoid space	Cisterna basalis
Passage through the dura mater	Foramen jugulare
Passage through the cranial base	Foramen jugulare
Innervation areas	**motor:** pharyngeal muscles (cranial part), M. levator veli palatini, M. palatoglossus, M. palatopharyngeus, M. stylopharyngeus **sensory:** mucosa of the pharynx (cranial part), Tonsilla palatina, posterior third of the tongue, Plexus tympanicus, Membrana tympanica (inner surface), Sinus caroticus **special sensory:** tongue (posterior third) **parasympathetic:** Glandula parotidea (via Ganglion oticum), Glandulae linguales (posterior)

60.10 N. vagus [X]

Nuclei (quality)	• Nucleus ambiguus (SVE) • Nucleus solitarius (SVA, GVA) • Nucleus dorsalis nervi vagi (GVE, GVA) • Nucleus spinalis nervi trigemini (GSA)
Exit point from the brain	Medulla oblongata: Sulcus retroolivaris
Location in the subarachnoid space	Cisterna basalis
Passage through the dura mater	Foramen jugulare
Passage through the cranial base	Foramen jugulare
Innervation areas	**motor:** pharyngeal muscles (caudal part), M. levator veli palatini, M. uvulae, laryngeal muscles **sensory:** dura mater of the Fossa cranii posterior, deep part of the Meatus acusticus externus, Membrana tympanica (outer surface) **special sensory:** base of the tongue **parasympathetic:** organs of the neck, thorax and abdomen up to the CANNON-BÖHM point

60.11 N. accessorius [XI]

Nuclei (quality)	• Nucleus ambiguus (SVE) • Nucleus nervi accessorii (SVE)
Exit points from the brain	Radices craniales: Medulla oblongata: Sulcus retroolivaris → N. vagus [X] Radices spinales: Medulla cervicalis (lateral)
Location in the subarachnoid space	Cisterna basalis
Entry point into the cranial cavity	Foramen magnum (Radices spinales)
Passage through the dura mater	Foramen jugulare
Passage through the cranial base	Foramen jugulare
Innervation areas	**motor:** M. sternocleidomastoideus, M. trapezius (together with the Plexus cervicalis)

60.12 N. hypoglossus [XII]

Nucleus (quality)	Nucleus nervi hypoglossi (GSE)
Exit point from the brain	Medulla oblongata: Sulcus anterolateralis
Location in the subarachnoid space	Cisterna basalis
Passage through the dura mater	Canalis nervi hypoglossi
Passage through the cranial base	Canalis nervi hypoglossi
Innervation areas	**motor:** intrinsic muscles of the tongue, M. styloglossus, M. hyoglossus, M. genioglossus

Cranial nerves

61 Functional organisation of the isocortex: primary and secondary cortical areas

61.1 Primary cortical areas

Primary cortical areas*	Location	BRODMANN's area(s) (employing histological parameters, the cerebral cortex is divided into 52 cortical areas)
Primary somatomotor cortex	Gyrus precentralis, frontal lobe	4
Primary somatosensory cortex	Gyrus postcentralis, parietal lobe	1, 2 and 3
Primary gustatory cortex	inferior part of the Gyrus postcentralis (corresponds to the sensory cortical area of the tongue) parts of the Pars opercularis and of the insular cortex	43
Primary visual cortex	parts of the Sulcus calcarinus in the occipital lobe	17
Primary auditory cortex	Gyri temporales transversi (HESCHL's transverse gyri) of the Gyrus temporalis superior in the temporal lobe	41

*Not listed are the primary olfactory area (Cortex prepiriformis) and the numerous vestibular cortical areas of the isocortex.

61.2 Secondary cortical areas

Secondary cortical areas*	Location	BRODMANN's area(s) (employing histological parameters, the cerebral cortex is divided into 52 cortical areas)
Secondary motor cortical areas (pre-motor and supplementary motor cortex)	anterior to the primary motor cortex in the frontal lobe	6, 8
Secondary somatosensory cortex	posterior part of the primary somatosensory cortex in the parietal lobe	5
Secondary visual cortex	adjacent to the primary visual cortex in the occipital lobe	18, 19
Secondary auditory cortex	adjacent to the primary auditory cortex in the temporal lobe	42

*Only the most important secondary cortical areas are listed.

62 Nuclei of the thalamus (selection)

Group	Nucleus	Function
Specific sensory relay nuclei	Nucleus ventralis posterolateralis	sensory input from spinal nerves
	Nucleus ventralis posteromedialis	sensory input of the head and gustatory afferences
	Nucleus corporis geniculati medialis	part of the auditory pathway
	Nucleus corporis geniculati lateralis	part of the visual pathway
Specific motor relay nuclei	Nuclei ventrales anterior et intermedius	coordination of the cerebellum and basal ganglia of the motor system
Association nuclei	Nuclei pulvinares	integration of diverse specific sensory inputs
	Nuclei mediales	close relationship to the prefrontal cortex ('personality')
	Nuclei anteriores	part of the limbic system
Nonspecific relay nuclei	Nuclei intralaminares (centromedianus, parafascicularis)	parts of the reticular system, important functions for alertness and consciousness
	Nuclei mediani	sensory integration